# Communication in Midwifery: Theory and Practice

FIRST EDITION

# Communication in Midwifery: Theory and Practice

**TANIA STARAS, BA, MA, PhD, RM, PGCHE, FHEA**
Principal Lecturer in Midwifery
School of Sport and Health Sciences
The University of Brighton
Eastbourne, UK

ELSEVIER

**ISBN:** 978-0-323-88399-3

Printed in India
Last digit is the print number: 9 8 7 6 5 4 3 2 1

**Content Strategist:** Andrae Akeh
**Content Project Manager:** Taranpreet Kaur/Suthichana Tharmapalan
**Design:** Bridget Hoette
**Marketing Manager:** Deborah Watkins

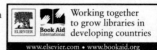

Working together
to grow libraries in
developing countries

www.elsevier.com • www.bookaid.org

# CONTENTS

I initially came up with the idea for this book in the winter of 2020 when the UK was in its second major COVID-19 lockdown. As a lecturer in midwifery, I, together with my colleagues, had pivoted to online teaching and student support in the first lockdown in the spring of 2020. This had already made me think about what and how we communicate. Out in the real world, we saw and heard what health professionals, including midwives and student midwives, were going through in continuing to give care to pregnant women and birthing people. At the same time, my daughter was pregnant with her first child and experienced her pregnancy journey through the lens of COVID. This included a minimal number of face-to-face appointments, undergoing all ultrasound scans and early labour admissions alone and being cared for by professionals in masks, visors and gowns. We talked a lot about how this made her and her partner feel about her pregnancy, birth and postnatal period.

The impact of the COVID pandemic continues to be felt both in care structures and in the memories of those who were on their child-bearing journey in the thick of it. It has impacted significantly on communication in maternity, but it was not the only factor that drove me to plan this book. There are a myriad of midwifery textbooks and online resources out there for students and practitioners to access. Many focus on the essentials of clinical care, others on specific aspects such as research or leadership. I felt strongly that there was a need for a book which put communication at its heart. I wanted a book which would highlight the skills and expertise that midwives have and help to pass this on to the next generation. But I was also aware of wider challenges to maternity care, of which communication was a huge part, and which needed addressing openly and honestly. We cannot shy away from the difficult conclusions reached by the Kirkup (2015) and Ockenden (2022) reports into maternity care which highlighted the traumatic and dangerous impacts of poor communication. Neither can we ignore areas of contemporary concern, including racism and unconscious bias in health care, including the maternity services, and the growing need to offer nongendered support to parents. The book addresses these issues in a practical way which helps us to move forward, whilst also acknowledging that debate around these issues continues.

It is something of a cliché to say that people remember the care given to them in pregnancy and labour and that even more pertinently they remember what was said to them—the throw-away remarks, the things that made them anxious or as though they hadn't been heard, the mistakes and the dismissiveness. But people also remember the good bits—the kindness, care, consideration and respect shown to them. I remember 25 years ago being told by a doctor that my planned home birth was risking my baby's life, just as I remember the midwife saying to me afterwards, 'it's your body and your baby—you will be fine'. That brief moment of connection, and the confidence it demonstrated in my judgement and my body, stayed with me. I continued with my plans and laboured and gave birth at home with no problems.

This book is intended to be a resource for anyone who is involved in care for women and other people in their child-bearing year. Obviously, the book is written with student midwives in mind, but its ideas and principles have much broader applicability than that. As a qualified midwife, support worker, administrator, doula, medical student or doctor, I hope you will find ideas in this book which are useful, thought-provoking and challenging. Similarly, if you work with women and people through charities or peer support groups, I hope you will find sections that help you in your work, and in the support you give.

Note on language: All contributors to this book support the principles of inclusivity, but we have chosen not to take a specific editorial line. In some places the terms 'women and birthing people' are used, but at others 'woman' can be taken to include people who do not identify as women but are pregnant or have given birth. Similarly, where the term 'parents' is used, this should be taken to include anyone who has main responsibility for caring for a baby.

*Tania Staras*
January 2023

# CONTRIBUTORS

**Cathy Ashwin** is a qualified midwife with a PhD in Midwifery. Her area of interest is in Public Health and counselling communication. She has worked within the community setting, including smoking cessation support for pregnant women and families. As a midwifery lecturer, she promoted the value of counselling and communication to her students within the wide range of subjects taught. Contributing to the collating and dissemination of research was included in her role as Head of Midwives Information & Resource Service (MIDIRS). MIDIRS is a source of information for midwives and allied health professionals in the form of a quarterly journal and an extensive collection of literature resources. Cathy is currently a freelance midwifery consultant and holds an honorary position with the University of Nottingham as assistant professor. She has published papers and contributed to several book chapters.

**Rebecca Brione** is a PhD student in Philosophy and Medicine at King's College London. Her current research aims to conceptualise harm in nonconsented and unwanted vaginal examination and to understand why it can be so difficult to successfully say no to examinations. She has a broad interest in consent and mental capacity during maternity care and coleads a research network on 'Narratives of consent and invisible women'. She has held advisory roles in major reproductive and maternity research programmes in the UK and is a lay examiner for the Royal College of Obstetricians and Gynaecologists. She previously worked for the UK human rights charity Birthrights.

**Katie Christie** is a qualified midwife with an MSc in Women's Health and a PGCE in clinical simulation and medical education. She currently works as a consultant midwife at University Hospitals Sussex NHS Foundation Trust. Her career has mostly been working clinically, specifically caring for women and their families in the intrapartum period. Katie has experience with working with different complexities and different birth settings as well as being a clinical leader within the maternity services. Other roles include leading the local professional midwifery team, working within the maternity education team alongside Brighton and Sussex Medical School (BSMS) and supporting women with cardiac disorders when birth planning. Her current work focuses on supporting women and people who choose to birth out of guidance.

**Jane Cleary** is a registered midwife and Professional Midwifery Advocate with a PGCert in Health and Social care. She currently works as a consultant midwife in Sussex. She set up a Birth Stories listening service in 2005 which has now become an integral part of maternity services. Since that time, she has been involved in working with women and families to support psychological wellbeing and care after birth trauma. She has worked as a practice development midwife/clinical skills facilitator and has ensured that women's/people's voices are heard within the learning for all professionals in maternity care. Jane received a Trust award for her innovation within training and development. Her current work involves advocating for women within midwifery to support their choice and decisions, recognising the importance of being listened to, understood and supported throughout their experience. She works closely with her midwifery colleagues in her advocacy role and continues to support them in their clinical midwifery work and career.

**Jo Gould** is a Registered Midwife, Senior Lecturer in Midwifery and Lead Midwife for Education at the University of Brighton. She teaches on the undergraduate Midwifery programme, with a focus on physiological labour and birth. Prior to qualifying as a midwife, Jo completed a BSc (Hons) in Architecture. She codesigned and jointly facilitates the 'Birth Space Project', a cross-disciplinary workshop with the School of Architecture focused on reimagining birth environments that better meet the needs of women, families and health professionals. She has published on midwifery education, midwifery knowledge and perineal management.

**Kate Levan** is a qualified midwife and professional midwifery advocate with 20 years of clinical experience. She currently works within the field of patient safety in a specialist role and has been doing so since 2014. Kate has a special interest in working with families and clinicians to achieve the best outcomes possible, and in promoting open and effective communication.

**Jane Rooney** is a qualified direct entry midwife and has worked across all fields of clinical practice in midwifery, specialising in providing enhanced care to vulnerable women, birthing people and families, with an interest in public health midwifery challenges. She has experience in clinical leadership, midwifery education, curricula and programmes, international midwifery and project leadership. Her current role as Head of Women's and Children's Health includes strategic networking and decision-making. Jane also has experience as a Lead Midwife for Education (LME), a statutory role concerned with quality assurance and maintaining midwifery education standards within the Nursing and Midwifery Council and higher education frameworks. She is also involved in research, including as a part-time doctoral student investigating women's narratives of negated childbearing throughout the continuum, and is currently writing up her research. Jane has an ongoing passion for public health midwifery, professionalism and communication and role modelling for the midwives of the future.

**Tania Staras** is a qualified midwife with a PhD in history. She currently works as a Principal Lecturer in Midwifery at the University of Brighton. Her teaching covers the range of the preregistration midwifery curriculum with particular expertise in research issues, sociology, social policy and professional issues. She has published extensively on the history of midwifery and maternity in the 20th century, including

*A Social History of Maternity Care*, published by Routledge in 2012. Her current work explores the development of policy and practice in maternity between 1960 and 2000, particularly narratives of risk and normality, the development and impact of technology, and the development of media in reflecting and 'selling' narratives of pregnancy and birth. *Note:* Tania has previously published as Tania McIntosh.

**Michelle Tant** is a qualified midwife, currently working as a Senior Lecturer in Midwifery at the University of Brighton. She started her journey into midwifery as a National Childbirth Trust Breastfeeding Counsellor in 2007, providing one-to-one breastfeeding support and facilitating antenatal infant feeding classes for expectant parents. She continues to do this privately in the local area. Her teaching at the university spans the preregistration midwifery curriculum with a particular focus on postnatal care, including infant feeding. She has published on topics including breastfeeding, resilience, bereavement and postnatal care and has a particular interest in social justice and feminism. Her current area of research is related to the professional socialisation of student midwives.

**Rebekah Wells** is a former NHS midwife with an MSc in Psychology and a PG Cert in Psychological Therapies Practice. She currently works as a Psychological Wellbeing Practitioner (PWP) in an NHS Improving Access to Psychological Therapies (IAPT) service and is a Graduate Member of the British Psychological Society (GMBPsS). Over the past two decades, she has worked extensively providing support to families in the transition to, or evolution of, parenthood, across a range of public, private and voluntary sector roles. She has a particular interest and expertise in perinatal mental health support. Rebekah has published papers in a variety of midwifery journals.

**Ray Wild** is a registered midwife, and lecturer at University of Derby. Ray mostly teaches nursing and midwifery colleagues who qualified in other countries to gain British degrees. Their midwifery practice focussed on healthcare injustice and service improvements in maternity care and the early years. Before becoming a midwife in 2010, Ray was a community development worker, and they believe that people with lived expertise are the best designers of care that works for them. Between 2016 and 2020, Ray worked locally and nationally on Continuity of Carer and supporting Black and Brown women's advocacy for an antiracist maternity service. Ray is currently researching trans people's experience of lactation and feeding their babies.

**Fawzia Zaidi** is a registered midwife and works as Senior Lecturer in Midwifery at the University of Brighton. She teaches across the preregistration curriculum with expertise in research, culture and diversity and obstetric emergencies. She has published widely and is a journal peer reviewer in these areas. Her PhD thesis used video elicitation methods and presented a theoretical model of decision-making of experienced midwives responding to obstetric emergencies. She is a Trustee for the Sussex Interpreting Service.

# ACKNOWLEDGEMENTS

A book like this is very much a collaborative endeavour. First and foremost, I would like to thank the chapter contributors who squeezed time out of their overloaded working lives to share their knowledge and experience. I have had a lot of conversations with my students about this book and its contents—these conversations have helped to shape how the book developed and what it contained. I would like to thank all my students, past and present, at the Universities of Nottingham and Brighton for teaching me as much as I have taught them.

All contributors to this book thank the midwives, doctors and support staff in clinical practice for their work, their insights and their wisdom. They have also helped to shape this book.

Finally and most importantly, we thank women, birthing people and families—keep being honest and open about what you need from maternity services and caregivers.

*Tania Staras*

# CHAPTER 1

# Introduction

Tania Staras

Modern midwifery can be rewarding, challenging and complex. In everything we say and do, in every encounter we have, communication matters. It has an impact on women's and people's physical and psychological wellbeing and it has an impact on how we work in teams and share ideas and information. Communication is at the heart of all practice because midwifery is based on human relationships. Kind, honest and open communication is vital in providing safe, person-centred care. This means that we talk, explain and show. It also means that we comfort, care, empower and, above all, *listen*. However, it can be challenging to ensure that this is what we offer to families. Busyness, under-staffing, professional hierarchies and defensive practice can all have a negative effect on what we communicate and how we communicate. When we get communication wrong it can have devastating consequences. On the other hand, when we get it right, communication has a hugely positive impact on safety, outcomes and wellbeing for families and babies. It is also the glue that holds the maternity services together; clear, respectful communication enhances how we feel about our role and how we make connections and build support for our professional practice. This book is another tool to help you in developing your knowledge and skills around communication in midwifery. It considers the theoretical and practical dimensions of communication and uses case studies to put ideas into real-world context and to give you ideas and strategies to take into the practice areas.

Communication is about more than exchanging information. The chapters in this book explore approaches to communication across different settings and consider the theoretical basis of communication, including ethical principles. Case studies and practical examples are used throughout to explore topic areas in ways which are thought-provoking, accessible and useful. These include communication in pregnancy, birth and the postnatal period and the use of written, verbal and non-verbal approaches. Complex scenarios where communication may be challenging are explored—examples include diverse groups, trauma and loss. New methods of communicating are considered, including the use of the internet and social media, and the benefits and challenges of these are explored. The importance of communication between professions is highlighted and ways in which this can be enhanced are explored. The book considers contemporary issues of consent, risk and safety in maternity care and explores the challenge of communicating complex ideas in meaningful ways. The intention of the book is to support midwives and others in thinking about and developing nonjudgemental communication strategies with a wide range of people. Particular attention will be paid to collaborative communication and communication with women and families in the light of the reports of Kirkup (2015) and Ockenden (2022), which highlighted the traumatic and dangerous impacts of poor communication. Other areas of contemporary concern include racism and unconscious bias in health care, including the maternity services, and the growing need to offer nongendered support to parents. The use of language and communication strategies in relation to these areas will be explored.

Above all this book supports students, midwives and everyone who works with people across the childbearing year. The book is designed to support you in thinking critically about communication and in enhancing your knowledge and skills. It will help you in navigating the nuanced and complex situations you encounter every day where clear, honest and collaborative communication is vital. It will support you to refresh and develop your theoretical understanding around communication and to build a practical toolkit of ideas and strategies for use in a range of settings and with diverse groups of people.

## How to Use This Book

The first thing to say is that this is not the kind of book which you will need to read from cover to cover (although you are more than welcome to do so!). Each chapter is designed to stand alone, and to give you theory and practice around different issues or points on the childbearing journey. Use the book to develop your understanding of the theory of professional communication or to dive into particular topics or look for ideas about developing your personal communication skills and practice. You might have come across an issue with communication during a booking appointment or in labour, for example, and want to use the relevant chapters in this book to explore it further. All the chapters will give you evidence-informed theoretical perspectives as well as ideas and strategies to take back into practice. As well as heading to the chapter which will help you with your assignment or practice issue, do also look at the other chapters. You will find a wealth of ideas, suggestions and discussion in all of them and you might discover something you were not expecting but which really resonates with you or sparks your thinking and practice development.

As you will see as you flick through the pages, this book does not expect you to plough through large chunks of text. In putting the book together, we have been mindful of how it might be used: to dip in and out, to find evidence or ideas around a particular issue or situation. We have tried to make sure that the book itself communicates its ideas effectively and practically. You will also notice that the book is not designed to be read passively. Scattered throughout the chapters are case studies, practice points, moments for reflection and activities for you to complete. Look at these as you read through the chapters. Decide if a particular activity is useful to you. Complete it however you wish—writing, sketching, audio recording or making a personal blog. The activities and reflections are designed to challenge your thinking and help you to build up your own personal toolkit of strategies for communicating with different people in different circumstances.

The chapters in this book have been written by different authors with expertise in different areas of midwifery practice, teaching and research. Although they are designed to be read as standalone chapters, you will see that each chapter has links to other chapters which you might also find useful or relevant for the topic you are exploring. This is because midwifery practice is so intertwined. Each chapter also ends with a short list of references and resources or further reading. The resource list for each chapter is annotated, so you will have some idea of what you might find when you follow a link and how it might further develop your knowledge and understanding.

You will also notice that there is some repetition of concepts and principles across the chapters. This is deliberate because each chapter will explore issues in a different way and through a different lens—topics will be covered using ideas and examples relevant to the chapter.

Finally, as with any book, this book is not the final word. It can only scratch the surface of concepts in communication. Practice in this area is dynamic—always developing and changing. We have tried to cover a wide variety of midwifery topics in a sensitive and thoughtful way but ideas and beliefs around communication will continue to change. Use the exercises in the book, the resources and your own practice and reading to develop your knowledge and skills in midwifery communication. And always remember that good communication is not an optional extra in midwifery—it *is* midwifery.

## What You Will Find in This Book

The chapters in this book are arranged in four main themes. The first theme covers *theories and concepts*, the second looks at *responsive communication*, the third covers *communication in practice* and the final one looks at *professional communication and personal development*. Here, you will find a brief outline of the chapters relating to each theme. This will help you to navigate the book.

### CHAPTER 2: ON THE RECEIVING END: THE SERVICE USER'S PERSPECTIVE

This chapter sits before the thematic section because it is designed to remind us exactly what midwifery communication is for. This chapter puts people and families at the centre of communication in maternity by exploring the service-user perspective across the childbearing year. Remember the principles expressed in this chapter as you work through the more academic and professional chapters.

## Part 1: Theories and Concepts

The chapters in this section set the scene by exploring what communication is, how we can use it as midwives and some of the challenges in communicating complex ideas such risk.

## CHAPTER 3: PRINCIPLES OF COMMUNICATION

This chapter sets the scene much more broadly by exploring what we mean by the idea of 'communication' in general. We will look at ways of communicating and consider the reason it is fundamental to us as humans in both an individual and a social context. The chapter will then consider what specific meanings and attributes communication has across midwifery practice. We will consider what **good and bad communication** looks like and the impact that this might have on us, families and the service. The chapter then briefly sketches the **history of communication** in childbirth and looks at its role in the sociology of health. This allows us to put into context the attributes of midwifery communication and explore some of challenges to effective communication. Finally, we will consider what **professional codes** such as that of the Nursing and Midwifery Council (NMC) expect of midwives in relation to communication.

## CHAPTER 4: THEORIES OF COMMUNICATION AND COUNSELLING

This chapter explores some **models of communication** and considers how we might use them in midwifery practice. We will then look in detail at **counselling skills** as a particular type of communication that midwives use daily. This chapter explores communication within a counselling situation and offers both **theoretical** and **practical approaches**. In so doing it offers a deeper understanding of the nuances of the midwife–service user relationship and the effect this may have on the long- or short-term outcomes. Finally, a further area that cannot be overlooked is the preceptor–student relationship, where again there is a need for excellent communication skills and on occasion the counselling skills that may be required to support students through training and beyond into their professional career.

## CHAPTER 5: COMMUNICATING IDEAS

This chapter explores **health communication** and why it matters to midwives and other caregivers. It then explores the issues of **risk** and of **human rights** as they relate to the childbearing year. We then consider how we can communicate **complexity** and **uncertainty** to families and look critically at the strategies midwives use to explain or manage tricky issues. Finally, we take a brief look at **moral issues** and communication within the maternity services and consider to what extent we communicate ethically and honestly, even when we think we are doing the right thing.

# Part 2: Responsive Communication

The four chapters in this section take a broad thematic approach to communication issues across the childbearing year and with a range of diverse groups.

## CHAPTER 6: CULTURALLY COMPETENT COMMUNICATION

This chapter considers the provision of respectful, person-centred communication with childbearing women, people and their families from **diverse groups**. It will include the neurodiverse, those with sensory support needs, ethnic minorities and lesbian, gay, bisexual, transgender, queer, questioning (LGBTQ+) groups. It will critically explore how personal and structural biases within maternity services are expressed during communication and can be mitigated by developing and applying the main attributes that underpin intercultural competent care. Accordingly, it will demonstrate how development of the attributes of cultural **awareness**, cultural **knowledge** and cultural **sensitivity** can support midwives in their intercultural communication.

## CHAPTER 7: PUBLIC HEALTH

This chapter focuses on communication for one of the key roles of midwifery practice—supporting and delivering care around **public health**. This chapter considers the background to public health in midwifery and the key principles of communication. It will then use the example **of smoking cessation** to work through the range of communication techniques and tools which midwives can use to deliver and develop their practice. Although smoking is the example topic, the ideas and techniques are applicable to and useful in all midwifery public health encounters.

## CHAPTER 8: COMMUNICATION AND COMPLEX CARE PLANNING

This chapter uses real-world examples to explore some of the issues and challenges of planning and providing **complex care**. It begins by considering typical care pathways and ways we may need to adapt these to suit individual people. It then explores the importance of **multidisciplinary** communication before using case studies to explore examples of care, including **homebirth out of guideline, freebirth** and **medical/obstetric complexities**.

## CHAPTER 9: COMMUNICATION AROUND LOSS AND TRAUMA

This chapter will begin to explore communication around **loss and trauma**, starting by giving some thought to definitions and considering application to practice throughout. The nature of both loss and trauma as **unique and individually constructed** experiences will be discussed and the crucial role of individualised communication will be considered. Principles of confident, sensitive, respectful and clear communication will be elaborated on for application both in the midst of a loss or traumatic event and in the immediate aftermath. The role of **counselling and debriefing** in such situations will also be considered, and key skills for communicating with those who have had a previous experience of loss or trauma will be highlighted. Finally, the importance of communication for professionals in order to access their own support and debriefing will be explored.

# Part 3: Communication in Practice

Each of the chapters in this section includes case studies to highlight midwifery communication expectations, strategies and common issues. The principles explored in Parts 1 and 2 are embedded in these practice-focused chapters.

## CHAPTER 10: PREGNANCY

This chapter explores some key ideas about human communication and how it relates to everyday antenatal midwifery care. Sections will explore the **booking appointment, screening** and **birth planning**. The chapter will highlight the **continuity of care(r)** debates and the delivery of high-quality communication within the realities of 21st century care pathways and pressures on health care systems. It discusses communication between midwives and childbearing women and people; co-parents and wider support networks; and our colleagues in perinatal services and beyond.

## CHAPTER 11: LABOUR

This chapter provides a detailed exploration of communication in relation to **labour, birth and the immediate postnatal period**. Compassionate communication in early labour via **telephone triage** will be considered. Responsive verbal and nonverbal communication in established labour, birth and the immediate postnatal period will be explored. Communication and **informed consent** will be discussed. Finally, the chapter will consider communication related to **information exchange, handover and record-keeping**.

## CHAPTER 12: THE POSTNATAL PERIOD AND INFANT FEEDING

Responsive and person-centred communication is explored in relation to the **physical, emotional and physiological** transition to parenthood. This includes a discussion of the use of language around infant care and **infant feeding** and the significance of language and support relating back to the **birth experience**. We will be discussing some of the pressures on new parents to meet unrealistic expectations of the postpartum body about infant feeding and consider what role midwives have in bringing balance to this conversation. Finally, we will consider the emotional and psychological transition to parenthood and the impact of **birth trauma**, which serves to further reduce the 'bandwidth' of new parents' ability to adjust and adapt resiliently in the postnatal period.

# Part 4: Professional Communication and Personal Development

The chapters in this section focus on the individual midwife as a communicator at the bedside and beyond, including developing reflective and responsive practice.

## CHAPTER 13: COMMUNICATING WITH OTHERS

This chapter explores the principles and practice of communicating within and across the **multidisciplinary team**. It includes a discussion of **escalation** and managing **'grey areas'** (when a situation is not a clear emergency), **accountability** and **professional responsibility**. It also considers **record keeping** and the role and challenges of **handover**, where the goal is always clear, accurate information giving and planning. Finally, this chapter includes a section on responding to **complaints** and **investigations** and **raising concerns**. These are all areas which can be stressful to contemplate or be involved in, whether as a student or an experienced practitioner. This chapter gives practical ideas for managing our involvement in a way that supports honest transparent investigation and, ultimately, service improvement.

## CHAPTER 14: SPREADING THE WORD

This chapter explores how we can communicate with audiences beyond the bedside. Midwives are uniquely placed to tell stories of care, of birth and of their profession. This chapter considers who our different audiences might be and examines communication principles and strategies for reaching out to groups and individuals, including **students**, the **general public** and **academic or practice audiences**. Additionally, we take a critical look at **social media** and the opportunities and challenges of using these to talk about midwifery in a way which integrates our professional standards and regulations. Finally, there is a section exploring communication through **presentations, posters and writing** for publication. Writing, speaking and teaching about what we do can sometimes seem like a chore, but it can be creative, incredibly satisfying, fun and important.

## CHAPTER 15: REFLECTION, DEVELOPMENT AND CHALLENGES IN COMMUNICATION

This chapter puts your **professional and personal development** around communication centre-stage. The first section considers you as a practitioner, exploring what kind of communicator you are and what skills of communication you might seek to develop. The second section will examine how you can use **creative reflection**, support and **goal setting** to enhance your skills. It will suggest ideas and tools to help you in setting goals for yourself and working to embed communication skills and principles in a way that is meaningful and true to you and your practice. The final section will consider briefly some of the **challenges of contemporary practice**, including COVID-19, the future of midwifery and virtual communication.

## CHAPTER 16: CONCLUSION

A short conclusion draws together the themes of the book and highlights the learning and practice development principles. It reiterates the centrality of open communication to midwifery practice and care.

### References

Kirkup, B. (2015). *Morecombe Bay investigation report.* https://www.gov.uk/government/publications/morecambe-bay-investigation-report

Ockenden, D. (2022). *Ockenden report – Final: Findings, conclusions and essential actions from the Independent Review of Maternity Services at The Shrewsbury and Telford Hospital NHS Trust.* Her Majesty's Stationery Office (HMSO). https://assets.publishing.service.gov.uk/government/uploads/system/uploads/attachment_data/file/1064302/Final-Ockenden-Report-web-accessible.pdf

# CHAPTER 2

# On the Receiving End: The Service User's Perspective

Rebecca Brione

## Introduction

Women and birthing people remember the days on which they had their babies for the rest of their lives. They remember what was said. They remember how it was said. They remember whether or not they felt in control of the direction of their care. It may be just another day in the life to you, but the memories of those interactions will stay consistently with women and birthing people for years (Forssén, 2012; Simkin, 1991, 1992). As a midwife you have an immense power to shape those recollections through how you speak with, enwgage with and support every individual in your care.

This might be a pretty frightening way to start this chapter, but it needn't be. Each of you will have had your own reasons for entering midwifery. I imagine that for many, the desire to be *with woman, with birthing person*, will have been an important part of that. You became midwives to provide good, kind and dignified care. Communication with women, birthing people and families provides an opportunity, every day, to practice and live the values that brought you into midwifery in the first place.

I recognise that you are working in a situation of intense pressure. I realise too that practising person-centred communication might feel particularly hard when teams and units are overloaded. If anything, though, these are the times when a little kindness goes the furthest and is most appreciated by the recipient.

This chapter will talk about communication from the perspective of women, birthing people and families.[1] By communication I don't mean only what is said, but how, with what tone and what body language. The chapter will of course talk about

---

[1]In the chapter I refer both to women and birthing people, and try predominantly to use 'woman/women' when it relates to individual women's experiences. However, one of the most crucial things you can do is to see the person in front of you for who they are, and I would suggest that everything I say in this chapter has particular pertinence for people who may not normally feel 'seen' in maternity services. Communicating that people are welcome, are seen as themselves and are respected is vital, and everyone's business.

the vital role of communication in ensuring that you have legal consent for each and every intervention or examination you carry out. However, communication is about much more than this. It lends shape and flavour to individuals' experience of care—a dismissive word in an early interaction can put a person off asking for what they needs or even wanting to engage at all. Good communication has the power to buttress and build a person's self-trust in their ability to make the right choices for them and their baby. It can show them that you really are *with them* and their family, supporting them with the care they need at that moment.

In this chapter, I explore different aspects of communication, from the woman or birthing person's perspective. I first focus on some of the more straightforward facets of communication, sited in the context of the everyday demands put on you— the tick lists, booking systems and the paperwork. In the second section, I explore the importance of collaborating with the woman or birthing person to create a sense of mutual trust. In the final section, I will take a step backwards and consider the impact of the broader systems and spaces you are navigating.

This chapter doesn't pretend to be a 'how to' of communication. I offer a view that I hope will complement the professional expertise presented in this volume—an alternative perspective if you like—born of many conversations with women and birthing people and the reading of many first-person accounts of birth. Most of all I hope to inspire you to think about how you can use your communication skills to provide the best care possible to women and birthing people.

## Beyond the Tick Box

There is an enormous amount that your communication is expected to do every day. A huge amount of functional communication—giving and exchanging information—occurs just to get the job done, the person booked in, the birth plan made, consent discussed. In this section, I will talk about the role that basic communication skills have in helping you to negotiate these demands in a way that goes beyond the tick box, such that you are able to really see the person in front of you and understand their needs.

'Seeing the person' is not a 'nice to do'. It is crucial to safe care and to positive experiences. You have information that you need to get across, but women and birthing people also have information about what they need and what they prioritise. You cannot do your job without this information. They may well have information that is pivotal to their safety and to that of their baby (e.g. Hall et al., 2018, p. 45), but they also come with their pregnancy as a part of their broader life. They come with needs that may well not map neatly onto the professional frameworks you work within. In this section, I will explore the communication skills you need to navigate these spaces.

## MOVING BEYOND THE FUNCTIONAL

### Listening

It sounds trite to say that it is vital to listen to women and birthing people and really hear what they are saying, but it is also true.

At the most basic level, listening to people means just that—hearing what they are saying, what questions they are asking and doing your best to answer those questions as openly as you can. Even these simple interactions have the potential to shape a person's engagement with care and their sense of whether their care will be personalised to their needs or more of a 'conveyor belt'.

When I booked in for my antenatal care, I wanted to know what the Trust's policy on induction of labour was. I was dismissed—not unpleasantly—and told that I could discuss that later on, if necessary, closer to the time. It would have taken a few short sentences to give me some headline information about what was standardly offered, and to reassure me that any decisions on induction would be my choice and supported by more detailed conversations with health carers. That would have helped assuage an anxiety that was pertinent to me at that time, and throughout that pregnancy. It would not have negated a need to have a personalised conversation later on if induction was recommended, but it would have given me reassurance, and also my midwife some information about the sorts of things that might be particularly concerning to me during my care. It might, time permitting, have presented an opening for a direct conversation about *why* I was asking that question and what I really wanted to know. (Did I actually want to know what the policy was? Or was I really concerned about a particular aspect of birth, for example?)

Even in an urgent situation, you can take a brief moment to focus on the person at the centre and to understand what they need in that instant.

### Imparting Information

Seeing the person in front of you also means making sure that you are giving information over in a way that is clear and coherent for that individual—using interpretation and language support if that may help, and making sure that you are aware of any accessibility requirements (for example, the use of lip reading, or accessible formats for written information). Again, this runs the risk of sounding obvious, but it is striking, talking to women and birthing people, how commonly they describe *not* understanding why a particular course of action was recommended. It is always difficult from the outside to know exactly what information was offered, and what was understood, but women frequently describe their care being led by what was 'safer for my baby' without necessarily having understood why it was safer, or feeling that they had an option to choose otherwise (Birthrights and Birth Companions, 2019, p. 29).

One key thing to bear in mind is *why* you are imparting information. Perhaps sometimes it will be one-way information (communicating the standard schedule of antenatal appointments, for example), but often the purpose of imparting information is to support the person in making a decision about their care. Whilst this is not a textbook on law and consent, it cannot be emphasised enough that it is impossible to extricate consent from communication. The law itself is clear that consent requires women and birthing people to be given information about treatment or intervention risks that are material to them (*Montgomery v Lanarkshire Health Board* (2015) UKSC 11 at 87). It will often be your role to impart this information. However, there is no possible way for you to know what is material, or significant, to the person without reciprocal communication.[2]

## Conversation

This means conversation. It means responding openly and honestly to questions that are asked of you. Women commonly describe being 'shut down' when they attempt to ask questions to help them to understand recommended care (e.g. Birthrights and Birth Companions, 2019, p. 29), and health professionals reacting with surprise when asked for more supporting information on their recommendations. Failing to answer women and birthing people's questions fully and respectfully amounts to withholding the information that individuals need to make decisions about what happens to their bodies during one of the most significant points of their life.

Women and birthing people's questions are also a crucial information source for you. They enable you to build a picture of what might be material or significant to the person in front of you, and therefore what further information, questions or topics you might need to explore in order to enable them to make choices in their care and give legal informed consent.

Good communication involves being alert to nonverbal as well as verbal signals. Research into antenatal consent conversations has shown how frequently women's signals are missed when the functional aspects of communication are prioritised by health care professionals. In one observational study, researchers commented that clinicians (including midwives) were so focussed on the clinical nature of the consultation and getting consent forms signed that they missed signs that women were unhappy with the proposed care, the tension in the room between women and partners, and the pivotal importance of certain nonclinical factors in women's decision-making (Nicholls et al., 2021, p. 6). In some cases, clinicians appeared to think they had consent for an intervention when they did not—in one example they had a signed consent form but the woman had no intention to attend for care. The researchers commented that in some 'highly time-pressured consultations, we

---

[2]For a helpful summary on what clinical guidance says that women and birthing people should expect from consent conversations, see Birthrights (2021). Whilst this blog post was produced with consent discussions with doctors in mind, the same principles apply to your interactions with women and birthing people.

observed HCPs who wanted to "get on" with the consultation leaving women visibly frustrated and disengaged' (Nicholls et al., 2021, p. 7).

At an extreme, failing to 'read' nonverbal signals puts clinicians at risk of carrying out nonconsented interventions (which potentially comprises battery in law). More broadly, it signals that the woman or birthing person's feelings and input are not valid, that the power to lead conversations and make decisions is with the health care professional. Not only does this pose a significant threat to building relationships of trust (see next section) but also it prevents you from identifying possible support needs for individuals and families in your care. If you are not paying attention to me, why would I confide in you?

## WOMEN READ THEIR NOTES!

At this point I would also like to draw your attention to the oft-forgotten part of functional communication—the maternity notes. It is possible that the move to electronic records may in some cases be shifting greater ownership and author-powers to women and birthing people. Regardless, the major point I would like to make here still stands: assume that women and birthing people will read their notes. Women and birthing people want to know what has been written about them. They want to know that their notes are accurate and reflect their understanding of what has happened—that they can be trusted.

The written word comes with particular dangers for the midwife–service user relationship. So many aspects of parenthood feel like they are open to moral judgement or scrutiny from others—and pregnancy is no exception. The way in which an individual's decisions are recorded can be read as having moral weight that wasn't intended when the note was made. It is important both to be accurate and also to think about the language that you use in writing—always assume it will be read back by the woman[3], and think carefully about avoiding language that could be read as implying a judgement on her decision. I am still haunted by a comment written in my postnatal notes concerning breastfeeding. I doubt it was intended as disparaging, but over 10 years later I can still feel the embers of the visceral reaction I had at the time.

## CHALLENGE POINT: WHO DO YOU STAND FOR?

So far, we have looked at some of the functional aspects of midwife communication from the perspective of those on the receiving end. I have focussed on really seeing

---

[3] For more about humanising language, see Mobbs et al. (2018). For an excellent breastfeeding-focussed resource looking at how language can be heard as moralising even when this isn't intended, please look at the website *Feeling Good About How We Feed Our Babies* (Woollard et al., 2019).

the person in front of you, and briefly indicated the hidden messages of power that can be read into communication. Before we move on, I would like to ask you to step back for a moment and think about this some more.

Ask yourself: when you are communicating, particularly about choices or consent, who do you stand for? You are in a maternity setting to be with women and birthing people, yes, but you are also an employee. You are a member of a team of midwives. You have a professional registration to protect and a practice scaffolded by regulations, expectations and guidelines. How do those different factors shape how you communicate? Where does the power lie?

It is well recognised that midwives can feel pulled in different directions by these different calls on their professionalism, especially in situations where a woman or birthing person wants something outside standard guidelines or institutional practice (Feeley et al., 2022, pp. 3–4; Newnham & Kirkham, 2019, pp. 2153–2154). When you are in this situation, are you truly engaging in conversations to support the person in informed decision-making, or is there an element of directing them towards particular care choices that are more readily supported in your unit? There can be a thin line between providing information to make sure someone is making a fully informed choice and coercing or frightening them into care—for example by repeatedly checking that they understand certain risks involved in their decision (Birthrights and Birth Companions, 2019, p. 35) or asking their partner if they support the decision. It can be easy to inadvertently suggest that actually a person's choices are *not* valid, and that they don't get to choose, as in the case of the woman who declined vaginal examinations only to be told 'Why? That's ridiculous. We all need to do them' (Birthrights and Birth Companions, 2019, p. 34). What are the chances of that person feeling confident to assert their choices another time?

When you provide care that is truly person-centred, you place the power to choose with them and you contribute to building mutual relationships of trust. I will talk further about the specific role of communication in building these relationships in the next section.

## Getting to Know You

Good relationships and communication are intimately entwined. We all value a kind word, a friendly face and someone to talk to. In the context of midwifery, however, there is a much more fundamental reason to focus on using your communication skills to build relationships: these relationships are crucial to buttressing women and birthing people's autonomy, and confidence in their own decision-making. They also play a vital role in creating conditions which safeguard women and birthing people's emotional and physical safety—partly through sharing of information, but particularly through building relationships of trust. In this section, I will delve further into the roles of communication in shaping your relationships with the individuals in your care, creating the space for people to make decisions about their care that are right for them.

## CONTEXT: CREATING COMMUNICATIVE SPACE

In the previous section, I talked about some of the basics of communication, noting the need to think about what information you are sharing and why, and the importance of being alert to nonverbal signals. So, how do you create communicative space for women and birthing people to talk about what they need?

This may be easier in some situations than others. Time and continuity of relationship will often be beneficial. You will not always have these relative luxuries. However, researchers on the observational study suggest that, at a minimum, opening a consultation with questions such as 'what matters to you most?' can help shift the framing of discussions (Nicholls et al., 2021, p. 1). It may be helpful to specifically ask about nonclinical factors as women and birthing people may fall back on clinical framing as a presumptive 'appropriate' way of presenting the decisions they want to make or discuss.[4]

It is also worth thinking about some basics—are you showing that you are listening and taking the person in front of you seriously? Your body language talks. Most of us have been at parties where we just know that the person we're talking to isn't *really* listening—maybe they're looking over our shoulder for someone more interesting or just aren't fully present. We know. So do the women and birthing people in your care. No one will 'really want to open up' and be honest with you if you're not showing that you want to hear what is important to them and are prepared to engage with it (Birthrights and Birth Companions, 2019, p. 41).

## MORE THAN JUST A HEADLINE

At this point, I want to point to a possible trap that it is easy to fall into. I have already noted that clinical framing can easily dominate conversations. However, some people describe risk—whether clinical or social—dominating their entire care experience. Whilst I would not presume to tell you to ignore factors which may be important to a person's care, no woman or birthing person is ever 'just a headline' (Birthrights and Birth Companions, 2019, p. 64).

Unfortunately, women frequently describe being treated in this way. One doula and birth researcher wrote in her blog that 'I didn't experience antenatal care as a pregnant woman, but as "walking/talking diabetes"' (Horn, writing in Thaels, 2021).

---

[4]This may be particularly the case where the clinical discussion is focussed on the baby's health or outcomes (Coxon, 2014, p. 486).

Women with disabilities report being categorised as 'high risk' without anyone explaining why (Hall et al., 2018, p. 42), being told outright that they were a 'a health and safety risk' (Hall et al., 2018, p. 26) or feeling that they and their families were the subject of prurient interest (Hall et al., 2018, p. 35). Women describe this as explicitly dehumanising: 'You're not a pregnant woman you're just a body, because [sic] if I was a person to them, if I was a pregnant woman they would have read my file' (Hall et al., 2018, p. 53).

It is also worth pointing out that some women and birthing people—for example, those who are under the remit of services such as mental health care or social care—may be 'highly attuned' to potential judgement in how they are treated, spoken to and touched (Birthrights and Birth Companions, 2019, p. 61; Cardwell & Wainwright, 2018, p. 18).

Being seen—or being afraid of being seen—as a 'single story' (Birthrights and Birth Companions, 2019, p. 65) stands directly in the way of being able to build a relationship of trust, something that matters a great deal to women and birthing people (Nicholls et al., 2019, p. 6). Indeed, being able to trust your midwife can sometimes be 'more important than the detailed ins and outs of any proposed intervention' (Nicholls et al., 2019, p. 6; also Feeley et al., 2020, p. 11). This was certainly my experience: when I felt seen and heard as *me* by my midwife, then I was prepared to follow her advice because I trusted that she was making that recommendation in the light of knowing what mattered to me, and why.

## CURATING TRUST

So what do I mean by curating trust? I mean building a mutual trust, where the woman or birthing person trusts you and your care, and *you trust them and their experience.*

Communicating that you trust the woman or birthing person, their judgement and their decision-making is vital to supporting autonomy. This idea comes from feminist theorists of autonomy, who argue that individuals' decisions are shaped by the social and cultural networks they are in (such as family, friends and health care cultures) and that individuals' decision-making capacity can be shaped, enhanced or limited by those networks (Westlund, 2009, p. 42). Some argue that self-trust—that is, a person's ability to trust her 'capacity to make appropriate choices, given her beliefs, desires and values' (McLeod & Sherwin, 2000, p. 262)—is a particularly important part of autonomy. They argue that a woman's self-trust is, at least to some extent, at the mercy of those around her: an agent's 'trust in herself exists in part because others reinforce that trust in their relationships with her' (McLeod & Sherwin, 2000, p. 265). Put simply, a woman surrounded by people who doubt her decisions may be far more likely to question whether she has made the right choice.

Applied to the maternity care setting, this means that supporting a woman or birthing person's autonomy requires you to show and communicate that you trust her to make the right choices. It means showing that you value their knowledge of their pregnancy and their body. You cannot foster self-trust in someone if you doubt when they tell you they are in pain or in labour, or when they tell you they know what they need (e.g. Hall et al., 2018, p. 45). Women or birthing people whose knowledge of their bodies isn't believed experience this as profound distrust or even gaslighting (Cohen Shabot, 2019, p. 15). Women of colour are particularly prone to being distrusted or disbelieved (e.g. Awe, 2020; Bell, 2019).

How do you curate and support mutual trust? Again, by listening to women and birthing people, taking them seriously and responding to what they say. Feeley et al. (2020) call this 'listening to understand' (p. 9). You then need to move beyond communication to *action*, being willing to be creative to meet individual needs. In the study by Hall et al. (2018), women suggested midwives should 'Think "can do"', and 'figure out how to help' (p. 28) (also Feeley et al., 2020, p. 10). Putting commitments in writing may sometimes help to demonstrate a whole team's 'commitment' to such personalised care (Feeley et al., 2020, p. 13). *Show* that you trust through your speech, your body language, your reactions and your individual and team actions.

## CHALLENGE POINT: LEARNING TO SIT WITH DISCOMFORT

So far, so idealistic? But what about if you *don't* trust the person in front of you? Or if you are fundamentally concerned about the decision they are making?

I can here reiterate some principles of consent and good care, such as the fundamental right of women and birthing people to make the decisions they think are right, your role in supporting this and the need to expunge the words 'not allowed' from your vocabulary. However, I recognise that a commitment to these principles does not guarantee absolution from feelings of 'personal or moral discomfort' (Feeley et al., 2020, p. 3), which may be profoundly unsettling and make you want to 'turn away' or 'disengage' (Chadwick, 2021). Sometimes the discomfort may be a symptom of a particular situation; in others it could be as a result of feeling 'helpless' in the face of inequalities (Chadwick, 2021).[5]

Sometimes there may be things you can do to address your own discomfort— perhaps seeking support from a colleague or another service, finding further information or training on something that worries you or seeking reflective supervision. Some skills—such as 'not shy[ing] away from difficult conversations' (Birthrights

---

[5]Chadwick writes about thinking about the meaning of discomfort in research encounters as an important tool in working towards social justice (2021), but I think reflecting on discomfort, reasons for it and our possible responses can be a helpful practice in multiple situations.

and Birth Companions, 2019, p. 63)—may build up with practice. Relationships of trust enable you to be open with women and birthing people if you have concerns about aspects of their care, and to, for example, build plans which feel safe all round, based on in-depth 'understanding of what [individual] women needed' (Feeley et al., 2020, p. 12, see also pp. 13–14).

However, I suggest that there is also benefit in learning to 'sit with some uncomfortableness' (Birthrights and Birth Companions, 2019, p. 63). It is asking too much for care at such a fundamental moment of a person's life to always be comfortable, always feel safe. There will always be situations which feel difficult for you, decisions that worry you, and it is important that you are able to manage this ambiguity without looking to persuade or 'manage' women or birthing people into situations that feel safer for you, but may not for them.

This may be easier in some circumstances than others. In the final section, I turn briefly to your wider working context, communication within it and the mood music that this creates.

## Shaping the Mood

So far, this chapter has largely considered individual-level interactions, albeit with some recognition that they are shaped by your working environment and professional context. In this final section, I will reflect briefly on the way that this broader context can directly and indirectly shape communication with women and birthing people, and make it easier—or harder—to enact what this chapter has discussed.

### THE THINGS WE OVERHEAR

The maternity unit is not a quiet place. Communication happens all around—between reception staff and new arrivals, between members of the multidisciplinary team in the labour room or between colleagues chatting about a tricky situation. There may be little distinction to be made between what is said *to* a woman, *about* a woman or *near* a woman. This may be particularly pertinent on a ward, but I have experienced clinic setups where privacy was illusory at best, and I am sure you can think of similar examples from your own experience.

A lack of privacy can be a profound inhibitor of trust and safety, isolating and shaming women and pregnant people (Cardwell & Wainwright, 2018, p. 19). It also means that women and pregnant people hear what is said about them: if you have heard disrespectful comments made about a woman, her choices or her circumstances, then there's a reasonable chance she—or her partner or family—has heard those comments too (e.g. Gadsden, 2020a). Women report differential treatment on the basis of race from being able to hear that they were denied support that another woman was offered (Gadsden, 2020b). It is immeasurably harder to ask a woman to trust you, however good your own communication is, if the broader environment is telling her to question what is going on out of earshot.

## SITUATIONAL CHALLENGES

Dealing with these situational challenges is difficult because it involves acknowledging that there are influences on your communication that might feel beyond your control. To a certain extent, they *are*—you can't manage what other people say. However, you can consider what you contribute to the broader culture.

I say this knowing that this is difficult. You may feel you have very little power over the culture of a unit, especially in the earlier stages of your career. You may be working within rigid hierarchies and embedded ways of working. And we all end up taking communicative short cuts with colleagues who share a professional language.

You can, however, reflect on how these practices, norms and cultures impact on the communicative culture. You can identify where you have the greatest power to influence. When you are new to a workplace, you have a great deal to bring by asking *why* things are done a certain way. You can model the communication you would want to receive at every point in your career. Always keep in mind that however vulnerable you may feel doing this, women and birthing people are in a more vulnerable position. You know your way around the systems, environment and culture you are working in. They—often—will not. You may not feel that you individually have a great deal of power, but you do have power, and you have the responsibility to use that to contribute towards creating respectful and caring communicative environments.

## CHALLENGE POINT: STEPPING FORWARDS

Sometimes using your power responsibly means doing a difficult thing. In previous sections, I have challenged you on how you engage with things that feel difficult or uncomfortable on an individual level. Challenging you to step forwards amongst colleagues may feel more difficult still.

Throughout this chapter, I have described examples where women and birthing people felt that they were not respected, not heard and not trusted during their care. In this final challenge I want to ask: have you been in that room? Have you heard uncomfortable, disrespectful or downright discriminatory comments and stayed quiet? Have you stepped back when you could have spoken up?

I don't ask this to make you feel guilty. We are all human. But I do ask you to think carefully about this. In many situations you will not be the only person in the room. Maybe someone else will step forwards—or maybe they won't. It can take only one voice—yours—to disrupt a narrative or an exchange which may feel very uncomfortable for lots of people around you—not least the birthing person and their family. Even if you don't manage to make a difference in a particular scenario, it can make a big difference to a woman or birthing person to know that they had you as an advocate, supporting them and their interests. In investigative scenarios a midwife's testimony supporting a woman or birthing person may make it more likely that their account will be taken seriously (Brione, 2020, p. 35).

If you can think of times when you didn't speak up or were not heard, what can you learn from them? What strategies can you develop to help you next time? What can you do to create and maintain a professional community and culture that is shaped around individuals, their wishes and their choices? This book will give you much food for thought, but for the moment I would like simply to plant the idea that speaking up is a fundamental and hugely valued part of being 'with woman, with birthing person', as a friend, supporter and advocate. It is an essential part of living the values of midwifery.

## Concluding Thoughts

In this chapter, I have outlined one perspective on communication, honed from personal experiences, those shared with me and from a number of years immersed in advocacy and research around women and birthing people's experience of care. My own experiences include having 'gold standard' relationships of mutual trust and support, which I would wish for everyone, and—at different times—feeling dismissed, belittled, distrusted and left confused and distressed at points of intense vulnerability.

In this chapter, I have asked you to really *see the person* in front of you. To see them as an individual with a life narrative of which their pregnancy is a hugely important part but is not the only part. I have asked you to 'listen to understand' and to make sure that the information you give is clear and meets the woman or birthing person's needs. I have suggested that you cannot do this without a *conversation*, and without being alert to both verbal and nonverbal cues. I have suggested that you need to think about how to *create space* for the woman or birthing person to share with you and make sure you show you see them as *more than just a headline*. I have talked about the vital role of *curating trust* in caring for women and birthing people as the law requires—in supporting consent and individual decision-making. And I have highlighted some situations in which you may need to pay particular attention to creating trusting relationships. Finally, I have asked you to think about the broader communicative environment, in the clinic, on the ward and your role in building and sustaining this.

I have also posed challenges. I have asked you to think about *who you are standing for* in your communication with and care of women and birthing people. What do your interactions say about where decision-making power lies? I have suggested that you may need to learn how to *sit with discomfort* and develop strategies to support you with that. And in the final section, I have asked you to think about whether and how you *step forwards* when you hear things that are uncomfortable, disrespectful or even discriminatory. Fundamentally I have asked you to think about how you can play a maximal part in creating individual and cultural environments that are physically and emotionally safe and that let you live out the values of 'with woman or birthing person' or person-focussed care.

Women and birthing people know that your job isn't easy. We have a huge respect for the work you do, and enormous appreciation for the kindness, support and care that you bring. Above all, this chapter aims to help you practice in the way that you want to: with women and birthing people at the centre of their care.

### *References*

Awe, T. (2020). Black women are not listened to in labour, and our pain is not taken seriously. *Hysterical Women blog.* https://hystericalwomen.co.uk/2020/09/16/fivexmore-black-women-not-listened-to-in-labour-pain-not-taken-seriously/ [Accessed 10 January 2022]

Bell, P. (2019). *I kept saying 'I'm in pain, this isn't a joke' – then everyone looked shocked when my daughter popped out. i news.* https://inews.co.uk/opinion/comment/i-kept-saying-im-in-pain-this-isnt-a-joke-i-felt-completely-ignored-during-childbirth-268628 [Accessed 10 January 2022].

Birthrights. (2021). *Birthrights and GMC – What does informed consent mean in maternity care?* Birthrights. https://www.birthrights.org.uk/2021/09/17/birthrights-and-gmc-what-does-informed-consent-mean-in-maternity-care/ [Accessed 24 January 2022].

Birthrights and Birth Companions. (2019). *Holding it all together: Understanding how far the human rights of woman facing disadvantage are respected during pregnancy, birth and postnatal care.* London.

Brione, R. (2020). Non-consented vaginal examinations: The birthrights and AIMS perspective. In C. Pickles & J. Herring (Eds.), *Women's birthing bodies and the law unauthorised intimate examinations, power and vulnerability* (pp. 25–38). Hart Publishing.

Cardwell, V., & Wainwright, L. (2018). *Making better births a reality for women with multiple disadvantages.* Birth Companions and the Revolving Doors Agency.

Chadwick, R. (2021). Reflecting on discomfort in research. *LSE.* https://blogs.lse.ac.uk/impactofsocialsciences/2021/02/24/reflecting-on-discomfort-in-research/ [Accessed 10 January 2022].

Cohen Shabot, S. (2019). Amigas, sisters: We're being gaslighted. In C. Pickles & J. Herring (Eds.), *Childbirth, vulnerability and law exploring issues of violence and control* (pp. 14–29). Routledge.

Coxon, K. (2014). Risk in pregnancy and birth: Are we talking to ourselves? *Health, Risk & Society, 16*(6), 481–493.

Feeley, C., Downe, S., & Thomson, G. (2022). 'Stories of distress versus fulfilment': A narrative inquiry of midwives' experiences supporting alternative birth choices in the UK National Health Service. *Women and Birth, 35,* e446–e455.

Feeley, C., Thomson, G., & Downe, S. (2020). Understanding how midwives employed by the National Health Service facilitate women's alternative birthing choices: Findings from a feminist pragmatist study. *PLoS One, 15,* e0242508.

Forssén, A. S. K. (2012). Lifelong significance of disempowering experiences in prenatal and maternity care: Interviews with elderly Swedish women. *Qualitative Health Research*, *22*(11), 1535–1546.

Gadsden, S. (2020a). Get a takeaway for sepsis. *They Said to Me*. https://www.theysaidtome.com/get-a-takeaway-for-sepsis/ [Accessed 28 January 2022].

Gadsden, S. (2020b). Clear racism. *They Said to Me*. https://www.theysaidtome.com/clear-racism [Accessed 28 January 2022].

Hall, J., Collins, B., Ireland, J., & Hundley, V. (2018). *The human rights and dignity experience of disabled women during pregnancy, childbirth and early parenting*. Centre for Midwifery Maternal and Perinatal Health, Bournemouth University.

McLeod, C., & Sherwin, S. (2000). Relational autonomy, self-trust, and health care for patients who are oppressed. In C. MacKenzie & N. Stoljar (Eds.), *Relational autonomy: Feminist perspectives on autonomy, agency and the social self* (pp. 259–279). Oxford University Press.

Mobbs, N., Williams, C., & Weeks, A.D. (2018). Humanising birth: Does the language we use matter? *The BMJ Opinion*. https://blogs.bmj.com/bmj/2018/02/08/humanising-birth-does-the-language-we-use-matter/ [Accessed 10 January 2022].

Montgomery v Lanarkshire Health Board [2015] UKSC 11.

Newnham, E., & Kirkham, M. (2019). Beyond autonomy: Care ethics for midwifery and the humanization of birth. *Nursing Ethics*, *26*(7–8), 2147–2157.

Nicholls, J., David, A. L., Iskaros, J., & Lanceley, A. (2019). Consent in pregnancy: A qualitative study of the views and experiences of women and their healthcare professionals. *European Journal of Obstetrics & Gynecology and Reproductive Biology*, *238*, 132–137.

Nicholls, J. A., David, A. L., Iskaros, J., Siassakos, D., Lanceley. A. (2021). Consent in pregnancy – an observational study of ante-natal care in the context of Montgomery: all about risk? *BMC Pregnancy and Childbirth*, *21*(1), 102.

Simkin, P. (1991). Just another day in a woman's life? Women's long-term perceptions of their first birth experience. Part I. *Birth*, *18*(4), 203–210.

Simkin, P. (1992). Just another day in a woman's life? Part II: Nature and consistency of women's long-term memories of their first birth experiences. *Birth*, *19*(2), 64–81.

Thaels, E. (2021). Fighting for physiological birth in a 'high-risk' pregnancy. *Midwifery Unit Network*. https://www.midwiferyunitnetwork.org/fighting-for-physiological-birth-in-a-high-risk-pregnancy/ [Accessed 10 January 2022].

Westlund, A. C. (2009). Rethinking relational autonomy. *Hypatia*, *24*(4), 26–49.

Woollard, F., Trickey, H. Buchanan, P., Glowacka, M., & Dennison, L. (2019). *Feeling good about how we feed our babies*. https://feelingsaboutfeedingbabies.co.uk/. [Accessed 10 January 2022].

# PART 1

# Theories and Concepts

# CHAPTER 3

# Principles of Communication

Tania Staras

## Introduction

In the previous chapter we explored why good communication in midwifery care matters so much to women, pregnant people and families. Our role does not just revolve around our evidence-based knowledge or our clinical dexterity. How we talk and listen and act—how we are—is central to everything we do. Subsequent chapters in this book will explore communication in detail by focusing on particular episodes of care or complexities. This chapter sets the scene much more broadly by exploring what we mean by the idea of 'communication' in general. We will look at ways of communicating and consider the reason it is fundamental to us as humans both in an individual and a social context. The chapter will then consider what specific meanings and attributes communication has across midwifery practice. We will consider what good and bad communication looks like and the impact that this might have on us, families and the service. The chapter then briefly sketches the history of communication in childbirth and looks at its role in the sociology of health. This allows us to put into context the attributes of midwifery communication and explore some of the challenges to effective communication. Finally, we will consider what professional codes such as that of the Nursing and Midwifery Council (NMC) expect of midwives in relation to communication. These principles and expectations are relevant to every chapter in this book.

> **COFFEE BREAK ACTIVITY**
>
> Think about your day so far.
> - Who have you communicated with?
> - Why did you communicate?

# What Is Communication?

The word 'communication' comes from the Latin word 'communicare', meaning to share (Rosengren, 2000, p. 1) because it is the means by which we share knowledge and information. It is not specific to humans—animals and even plants share information about their environment and about danger and safety. For the purposes of this chapter, communication takes place between two people, or between groups of people. It allows us to reach common understandings about ideas and concepts, but also to disagree and argue.

Communication is one of those ideas that seem very simple because it is so much part of everyday life—we can't get by without it. At the same time, it is a slippery and complex concept that is hard to pin down simply because it is such an intrinsic part of life. At its most basic it is a way of transmitting and receiving information.

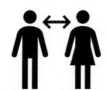

One person transmits information.
The other person receives it.

This doesn't just have to involve two people—it might be a class receiving information from a teacher or lecturer, for example.

However, communication is not as simple as transmitting your message and it being heard just as you transmitted it. Every time we communicate, we make spilt-second decisions about what we are going to say, how we are going to say it and what we think the person on the receiving end will understand by and do with our communication. And when we receive a communication, we make decisions about what we think the person transmitting meant to say, whether there were hidden meanings and what we want to do with the information—in other words we don't just accept the information, we interpret it. This means that communication is never a passive activity; even if we are just listening, we are engaged and involved. Equally if we choose not to listen or to ignore the information being transmitted that is still a decision we are making!

**QUICK REFLECTION**

Think about the last time you sat in a lecture or presentation.
- Did you feel interested/engaged? Why? If not, why not?
- How did the speaker share information—slides, hand-outs, talking?
- What techniques did they use to keep you interested—humour, storytelling, changes in speed and tone of voice, audience participation?

- How did you receive the information being transmitted—did you listen, take notes or daydream?
- Will you remember/use the information you received? Why? How? If not, why not?

## WHAT DO WE COMMUNICATE?

So far, we have used the word 'information' to convey what we are sharing. Communication is about far more than just 'information', however. Every time we communicate, we share our emotions, cultures and beliefs. We learn about the world, ourselves and others through expressing ourselves and through allowing others to express themselves. We begin to communicate from the moment we are born, seeking a connection with those around us. We communicate to tell people we are excited, happy, scared, anxious. In this way we share our ideas about what it is to be human and to feel. We also use communication in order to learn about society and our place in it. Communication and learning can be done formally through teaching and books, or it can be through informal storytelling, singing or dancing, or visual art. Communication is our social glue—it gives us a sense of who we are and of how we relate to others. Fig. 3.1 shows some of the broad underlying reasons for communication.

As we can see from Fig. 3.1, communication can be used to educate, to make connections with other people or to understand and position ourselves in wider society. It is also used to transmit ideas about power, whether that is a parent over a child, a teacher over a pupil or a governing group over a population. Communication is used to reinforce cultural and social beliefs and can be used to oppress or 'other' individuals or groups who are seen as different. In this way communication can be a tool for positive growth and understanding, but also a way of putting people down or disempowering them.

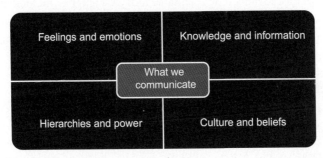

**Fig. 3.1**  What we transmit when we communicate.

TABLE 3.1 ■ **How We Communicate**

| Types of Communication | Examples |
|---|---|
| Preverbal/nonverbal | Touch, nonverbal sounds (grunts, screams, laughter), movement, dance, body language, facial expressions, eye contact |
| Verbal | Spoken words, singing, shouting, whispering, sign language, reading out loud, acting, storytelling, poetry |
| Read/written/paper based | Text, reading, writing, drawing |
| Mass communication | Radio, TV, Internet, newspapers, magazines, books, adverts, posters |

## HOW DO WE COMMUNICATE?

When we first think of communication we probably focus on the spoken or written word. But there are many ways to share the spoken and written word and, beyond that, many ways of communicating. Table 3.1 gives some examples of how we can *transmit*.

Remember as you look at this list, that communication also requires reception; think about how we receive each of these types of communication as a reader, listener or through touch. As we can see from this list, communication is not static. Both the *message* (what we communicate) and the *medium* (how we communicate) change over time and continue to evolve. When my grandmother was growing up before the First World War, written mass communication such as magazines was in its infancy, driven by growing rates of literacy in the UK. When my mother grew up, radio was popular—both for news and current affairs, but also for comedy, drama and music. In my childhood we had access to colour TV, and my daughter used a personal computer linked to the Internet from a young age. My grandchildren are learning to navigate communication through smartphones and social media. In the same way, the language and ideas that are acceptable or in popular currency change over time as society and culture evolve and develop. Many of the slang words I heard in the playground as a child would not be understood or acceptable today. Chapter 6 will look in more detail about communicating across cultural boundaries and with different groups, but it is vital to understand how dominant forms or styles of communication can have a disempowering and negative impact on groups and individuals.

### QUICK REFLECTION

At the beginning of this chapter, you thought about who you had communicated with today and why.
- Now go back to that activity and jot down how you communicated.
- Did you speak, write, listen?

- Did you use humour, raise your voice, offer explanations, instructions, or advice?
- Do you feel that you received what the other person/people were transmitting to you?
- Do you feel that the other person/people received what you were transmitting to them?
- What was easy about your communications?
- What was challenging?

'Effective communication between healthcare professionals and women is an integral component of safe maternity care …. Maternity services should foster a team approach based on mutual respect, a shared philosophy of care and a clear organisational structure for both midwives and medical staff, with explicit and transparent lines of communication'

OCKENDEN REPORT (OCKENDEN, 2022, P. 94)

## Why Does it Matter to Midwives?

As you have read the previous sections which discuss communication in general you have probably already begun to ponder how they relate to midwifery practice. As every chapter in this book reminds us, communication and midwifery are completely interlinked. It is obvious therefore that communication matters to midwives and that if we have an appreciation of the principles of communication then our practice and our relationship building will be more effective. Looking back at Fig. 3.1, we can begin to see how midwifery communication includes all the elements mentioned. Most obviously we impart **knowledge and information** to the people we are caring for. This can be clear factual information about appointment times or the physical process of induction of labour. It can also be more subtle—talking to people about how induction might make them feel and what they might experience in order to help them feel more prepared. The other sections in Fig. 3.1 are equally important. We communicate **the culture of maternity care and beliefs** through the way we talk about midwifery, by how we talk about pregnancy, birth and the new family, and by how we communicate with each other as professionals. In Chapter 5 we will look in more detail about how we communicate complex cultural ideas such as those around risk and uncertainty. In midwifery we are communicating not just clinical practice, but ideas as well.

It may seem obvious that we communicate **feelings and emotions**; the whole purpose of midwifery traditionally is to be 'with woman and birthing people', supporting and guiding. In many ways modern hospital-based technocratic models of pregnancy and birth have made expressing our emotions more challenging. We work to guidelines and protocols and there can be an expectation that we will solve problems and have all the answers. We are adept at receiving and perhaps managing the emotions of women and families, but we can struggle simply to accept peoples' feelings or to express our own in the context of our practice. Of course, it is not appropriate that our feelings are centre stage; we don't grumble about being tired or hungry in front of a labouring person. But it can be very powerful to express our humanity by sharing the joy of a birth, or the sorrow of a loss. Chapter 9 reminds us of the power of coming alongside grieving families and how this can have a positive impact at a challenging time.

The final area of communication highlighted in Fig. 3.1 is **hierarchies and power**. Many health systems are very hierarchical—this can be a useful way of managing very large and complex organisations. It also has significant implications for what practice looks like. This can be what different uniforms and badges signal about who is who. It can also be more subtle; a midwife cares for a labouring person. When the situation becomes more complex the midwife is required to call for medical opinion. This tiny moment demonstrates where the power and decision-making lie in that situation. Communication can also show that midwives can have power over women, even though we say we provide women-centred care which gives individual control and responsibility to labouring people. In reality in the hospital setting the woman is a 'guest'; the environment is unfamiliar as are the people, the rules and the expectations.

## Case Study

Woman and baby in postnatal bay. Person in uniform enters the bay and comes over to the woman.

*Woman:* Can you help me with feeding—he is struggling to latch on and I'm really stressed …

*Person in uniform:* I can't help you with that I'm afraid, I'm only here to do your obs. I will try and find the midwife for you.

*Woman:* Oh sorry, I thought you were a midwife.

*Person:* I'm just going to take your blood pressure …

*Woman:* Ok [holds arm out]. I had it done this morning …

*Person:* We do it every 4 hours—to make sure it's settling down. [Looking at the baby] She's lovely—look at that hair! Did you have heartburn?

*Woman:* He … and I didn't! I wasn't expecting so much hair!

## COFFEE BREAK ACTIVITY

Thinking about the sections in Fig. 3.1, can you find examples of where they occur in this conversation?

1. *Knowledge and information*
2. *Culture and beliefs*
3. *Feelings and emotions*
4. *Hierarchies and power*

Looking at the case study you may feel that not all reasons for communication are covered equally; very often one or two types will be more prominent. It can also be the case that the people having the conversation may feel that one type of communication is present and not be aware that others are also present in a hidden way. To take the example of the case study, the person giving care would probably say that **knowledge and information** around the care being given (in this case blood pressure) are the main features of the conversation. The woman might perceive that **hierarchies and power** are most noticeable—she wants help with feeding, but it is made clear that she can't have that but must do what the service requires, which is have her blood pressure taken. This gives the clear message that what she wants and needs is not as important as clinical guidelines, and therefore the power in the situation does not sit with her.

## GETTING IT RIGHT AND GETTING IT WRONG

Any communication between the professional and childbearing person is multifaceted and there is always more going on that just the words being spoken. We also know that women might not remember every detail of a conversation or experience, but they will usually remember how they felt and how they were made to feel. Thirty years after he was born, I remember suddenly being told at 39 weeks of pregnancy that my son might need to be born by C-section because his head was not engaged. I still remember how anxious, stressed and confused I felt when I left the room after my antenatal appointment.

When we get communication right, that is remembered—not always the detail but the feelings and emotions around the encounter. Of course, there is the issue of perception—we may think we have got it right, but the woman and family we are talking to may not feel that. Alternatively, we may not feel a particular conversation went well, but families felt positive about it. The next chapter talks in more detail about the process of communication, but it is always worth remembering to check back after any conversation—was any information given understood, have we left people feeling confused or uncomfortable, and how do we revisit the conversation to mitigate those feelings?

As the Ockenden Report (Ockenden, 2022) has highlighted, getting the basics of communication right is not a nice extra—it is absolutely key to the provision of good maternity care. Getting it wrong can have psychological and emotional consequences for families. It can also have clinical consequences if information is not understood or what women are telling midwives about symptoms or experiences is not heard or acted on. Kindness, compassion and really listening are as important as what we do.

# A Brief History of Communication in Maternity Care

When we communicate with women and families there are clear and obvious things we are communicating, such as information about an aspect of clinical care. But as we have already begun to explore, we are also communicating an array of other things even if we don't realise it. As we have seen, this can include beliefs, cultural ideas and assumptions about power and control.

This very brief section puts some of these issues in context by looking at the history of maternity care and its sociology. Obviously this can only be a snapshot, but it is designed to make some of our subconscious beliefs and ideas explicit. By developing our self-awareness around the underlying assumptions of our professional communication and relationships, we can work towards making them more open and meaningful.

One of the first things that UK student midwives learn is that 'midwife' means 'with woman' in old English. We build on this idea to see the midwife as part of a social view of childbearing, which puts the pregnant person at the centre of a network of relationships and the midwife alongside them. Historically in the UK midwives have always given support to the majority of births. Internationally, support figures, whether trained or untrained, have carried out the same role. The advent of medically trained professionals into the birthing room from the 17th century onwards changed the dynamic of care. In the UK they were exclusively men until the end of the 19th century and saw themselves as trained professionals when midwives were not (although medical training in obstetrics was rudimentary to say the least prior to the 20th century). Deliberately or otherwise, doctors seeking to gain a foothold in the lying-in room were extremely scathing of midwives who were their competition. An image of the midwife as dirty, ignorant, drunken and slipshod was spread by many doctors. In 1902 the first Midwives Act for England Wales was passed. This rehabilitated the image of the midwife but also left her (and it was always a 'her' before 1979 in the UK) subordinate to the doctor. Midwives were expected to focus on 'normal' or 'natural' cases, and doctors to take charge of emergencies or complex cases (McIntosh, 2012). This artificial division has led to some of the communication issues we see in contemporary practice. Doctors and midwives are expected to work closely together, but in practice have different philosophies and spheres of work. Despite having equal status to midwives as professionals, doctors are seen by the general public, and often by the structure of the NHS, as superior. This can cause challenges in effective and open communication. These relationships and the impacts on practice will be considered in more detail in Chapter 13.

The history of the relationship between doctors, midwives and childbearing women also impacts how communication takes place in contemporary practice. Before the mid-20th century in the UK, when birth primarily took place at home and people were paying for care, they had some control over the relationship between themselves and the professionals who cared for them. Even then, the communication did not always make for helpful care; sometimes women would have liked more support from midwives than they got, as this memory from a woman giving birth in the 1940s demonstrates: 'I was on nearly all night in labour and I told our Tony to go and get on his bike and get the nurse. She came and said "Oh, she'll be all night, I'm going home to get my ironing done"' (Smith, 1997, p. 48). As the woman commented ruefully, the midwife did not return until after the baby was born. Once birth moved into hospitals from the 1950s onwards the power in all relationships very much lay with the medical profession. Women and midwives were expected to be compliant and to accept that doctors knew best. Although this was gradually challenged by consumer groups such as the National Childbirth Trust from the 1960s onwards, for most women having a baby meant going into hospital and doing as you were told.

A significant shift came in 1993 with the publication of *Changing Childbirth*. This UK government report upended received wisdom about care around pregnancy and birth. Instead of putting the medical profession centre stage, with midwives playing a supporting role, it put women firmly in the picture:

> *The woman must be the focus of maternity care. She should be able to feel that she is in control of what is happening to her and able to make decisions about her care, based on her needs having discussed matters fully with the professionals involved.*
>
> EXPERT MATERNITY GROUP, 1993, P. 8

Themes of choice, continuity and control were developed which were designed to put women at the heart of decision-making. Effective communication was another, linked, element of the report. Some examples of the Report's objectives make this clear:

- *Women should receive clear unbiased **advice** and be able to choose where they would like their baby to be born.*
- *Women should have the opportunity to **discuss** their plans for labour and birth.*

- *The pattern of [postnatal] support should be appropriate to the woman's needs and planned in* **consultation** *with her.*

   *CHANGING CHILDBIRTH* (EXPERT MATERNITY GROUP, 1992)

Since *Changing Childbirth* the discussion has moved on, although the principles of working with families remain key. In *National Maternity Review*, 2016 also put communication at the heart of its mission, alongside kindness and safety. Over time the public have become less deferential towards and more critical of the NHS. As professionals, we must understand that our expertise and training do not give us the right to be rude, dismissive or patronising.

**QUICK REFLECTION**

- Do a very quick sketch of what a labour room of your experience looks like—it might be somewhere you work, or somewhere you have given birth.
- Draw the layout of the room and the main pieces of equipment in the room.
- How do you think a family might feel walking into this room for the first time?

The idea that the childbearing person should have agency and control over their body and their experience is not just linked to the history of maternity care. Challenges for communication can also be seen in the sociology of health and illness and what it means to be pregnant and give birth in our society. When birth took place at home and there was no antenatal care and very little postnatal care, pregnancy was seen generally as an altered but normal state. Labour was not necessarily seen as a special time, but rather as a disruption to everyday routines. In terms of how they remembered it therefore, women recalled getting on with things 'for half of my labour I did not realise that I was in fact in labour so carried on with my housework as normal' (Boyd & Sellers, 1982, p. 93).

The move to hospital for birth helped to change the idea of it. Hospitals were places for the sick—therefore the structures and systems of hospitals were designed around illness. On entering hospital, pregnant women were therefore encouraged by the set-up to see themselves as sick and to take on the role of patient. This meant wearing night clothes, lying in bed and returning to a childlike state of following orders. Women labouring in hospital were not expected to have any agency or even to consent to specific procedures. Being in hospital meant that control was handed over to professionals. An article in the consumer magazine *Mother and Baby* published in 1973 spelled out how unpleasant hospital birth could be with a 'Lack of privacy, emotional upset, failure to sympathise with the individual, parting from the family, husband and other children, and the conformity to rules and regulations are part of the price.' The price was a live baby, and effective communication was not seen as necessary (McIntosh, 2017).

Over time there have been efforts to make birth more personal and care more responsive and holistic. However, when exploring communication in midwifery, it is important to remember that memory and storytelling are important in how midwives, doctors and birth are seen today. When we communicate, we communicate our acceptance or rejection of some of these long-standing ideas about who has power, control and agency in the childbearing year. We must always bear in mind how essential it is to model inclusive supportive communication and really to come alongside pregnant people, rather than just playing lip service to these ideas whilst continuing to communicate our beliefs about the sick role or our professional importance.

## Professional Communication

So far in this chapter we have explored what communication is, why an understanding of the basic purpose of communication matters to midwives and considered some of the background to issues in professional communication. In this section we will focus on that concept of *professional communication* as distinct from communication between friends or in social circumstances.

### REGULATORY BODIES AND COMMUNICATION

The International Confederation of Midwives (ICM) sets out what it sees as core midwifery relationships, which are applicable globally:

> a. *Midwives develop a partnership with individual women in which they share relevant information that leads to informed decision-making, consent to an evolving plan of care, and acceptance of responsibility for the outcomes of their choices.*
> b. *Midwives support the right of women/families to participate actively in decisions about their care.*
> c. *Midwives empower women/families to speak for themselves on issues affecting the health of women and families within their culture/society.*
> d. *Midwives, together with women, work with policy and funding agencies to define women's needs for health services and to ensure that resources are fairly allocated considering priorities and availability.*
> ICM INTERNATIONAL CODE OF ETHICS FOR MIDWIVES (ICM, 2014, P. 1)

These principles all encompass elements of professional communication through information sharing, decision-making, empowering and working together. In the UK the NMC (2019) sets out specific midwifery skills and duties relating to communication:

*At the point of registration, the midwife will be able to:*

*1.11 use effective, authentic, and meaningful communication skills and strategies with women, newborn infants, partners and families, and with colleagues*

(NMC, 2019, P. 14)

Communication is highlighted as a core skill which cuts across all facets of midwifery practice:

6.1  *demonstrate the ability to use evidence-based communication skills when communicating and sharing information with the woman, newborn infants and families that takes account of the woman's needs, views, preferences, and decisions, and the needs of the newborn infant*

   6.1.1  *actively listen, recognise and respond to verbal and non-verbal cues*

   6.1.2  *use prompts and positive verbal and non-verbal reinforcement*

   6.1.3  *use appropriate non-verbal communication techniques including touch, eye contact, and respecting personal space*

   6.1.4  *make appropriate use of respectful, caring, and kind open and closed questioning*

   6.1.5  *check understanding and use clarification techniques*

   6.1.6  *respond to women's questions and concerns with kindness and compassion*

   6.1.7  *avoid discriminatory behaviour and identify signs of unconscious bias in self and others*

   6.1.8  *use clear language and appropriate resources, making adjustments where appropriate to optimise women's, and their partners' and families', understanding of their own and their newborn infant's health and well-being*

   6.1.9  *recognise the need for, and facilitate access to, translation and interpretation services*

   6.1.10  *recognise and accommodate sensory impairments during all communications*

   6.1.11  *support and manage the use of personal communication aids*

   6.1.12  *identify the need for alternative communication techniques, and access services to support these*

   6.1.13  *communicate effectively with interdisciplinary and multiagency teams and colleagues in all settings to support the woman's needs, views, preferences, and decisions*

   6.1.14  *maintain effective and kind communication techniques with women, partners and families in challenging and emergency situations*

> *6.1.15   maintain effective communication techniques with interdisciplinary and multiagency teams and colleagues in challenging and emergency situations*
>
> (NMC, 2019, P. 33)

These statements add up to a clear manifesto for professional communication. They remind us that the people in our care are not our friends but individuals and families to whom we owe a duty of care. We have a clear requirement to communicate compassionately, with care and kindness. We also need to be open and honest—when things go right and when things go wrong, when things are positive and when things are difficult or traumatic. We have a Duty of Candour which means apologising (without admitting fault) (Care Quality Commission (CQC), 2021). We should all work with families, supporting and empowering, and having the courage to say 'I don't know' in situations where the process or outcome may be unclear or unknown.

**COFFEE BREAK ACTIVITY**

Thinking about the relationship between midwife and client …
- What elements would you describe as 'friendship'?
- What elements would you define as 'professional'?

These principles apply whether we are a junior student or a senior manager, and they are not optional extras to good clinical care—they embed and embody our values as midwives, regardless of where and how we work.

## BEING A PROFESSIONAL FRIEND

We have indicated in the previous section that the midwife–family relationship is not one of friendship. However, in Walsh, 1999 studied the relationships which developed between women receiving care through a continuity of care model and their midwives. Women very much described their midwives as friends: 'I came to look upon Wendy (midwife) as a friend rather than a professional' (Sue; homebirth). That the midwife–person connection has elements of friendship dovetailed with elements of a more structured relationship which has led to it being described a 'professional friendship' (Pairman et al., 2006).

This is a change in emphasis from the mid-20th century when midwives were seen as set-apart from women by their professional status and power and treated with deference. Inevitably there are still aspects of this in communication with families, but the concept of 'friendship' embodies ideas of coming alongside, working with and empowering individuals. The 'professional' element reminds us that there should still be an appropriate and honest distance between the childbearing person and the midwife. This is for the simple reason that the relationship is very specific in time and space. We work to support and care for families in the childbearing year; it is not an open-ended evolving relationship. The relationship has a beginning, a middle and an end. This is true whether we work with families for 7 or 8 months in a continuity of care model, or whether we just support them for a few hours in labour or on the ward. One of the characteristics of an effective professional friendship is being able to bring it to a natural conclusion without distress on either side.

## PRACTICE POINTS

- Be open about the purpose and objectives of the relationship.
- Be clear that the relationship is time-limited and specific.
- Be clear about the ground rules of the relationship—what the boundaries are.
- Be flexible and able to renegotiate the relationship as circumstances change, e.g., the clinical situation.
- Be open, honest and trustworthy.
- Be respectful, kind and empathetic.
- Practice active listening in order to individualise the relationship.
- Remember that the childbearing person is at the centre of the relationship. Share your experiences if appropriate, but do not over-share.
- Be sensitive to your embodied power as a professional—think about how you present and how you share your knowledge and skills.
- Consider how to end the relationship in a supportive and empowering manner.

The concept of professional friendship can also usefully be applied to colleagues. In Chapter 14 we look in detail at midwife–student relationships, where the principles of professional friendship are clearly applicable. However, elements can also be helpful with colleagues generally; respect, openness and kindness but also the clear professional boundary setting can be helpful in maintaining effective working relationships.

## THE DOS AND DON'TS OF PROFESSIONAL COMMUNICATION

| Do | Don't |
| --- | --- |
| Be kind | Bully |
| Be honest | Patronise |
| Be trustworthy | Belittle |
| Be empathetic | Be paternalistic |
| Be friendly | Judge or moralise |
| Acknowledge the limits of your skill/knowledge | Make assumptions |
| Listen | Ignore |

Communication in midwifery can be complex. Relationships and situations change and we need to be responsive and flexible. If we prioritise always treating people as individuals rather than situations or problems, then that goes a long way to making our communication kinder and holistic. The Ockenden Report (Ockenden, 2022) has reminded us that above all else we need to be *humble*, to *listen* and to say *sorry* when necessary. Again, these principles can equally be applied to our working and professional relationships.

**QUICK REFLECTION**
- List five barriers to good communication in midwifery practice.
- How can we reduce their impact on care and relationships?

## BARRIERS TO COMMUNICATION

There are many barriers to communication in all walks of life. In relation to our professional practice they fall into different types. Some barriers are *philosophical*—our assumptions and beliefs as individuals and professionals may prevent us truly listening to pregnant and childbearing people. There are also *structural* and *organisational* issues—the busyness of the working environment and relationships among professional groups. There might also be *practical* barriers—language, for example. All the chapters in this book will discuss strategies for effective communication and ways around barriers and problems.

## PROFESSIONAL LANGUAGE AS A BARRIER

One of the first things we do as students in the maternity setting is try to get to grips with all the acronyms, Latin words and shorthand. If we understand what is being written and said, then we will begin to feel part of the culture and begin to develop our own sense of professional identity and connection. This socialisation into the midwifery role is vital, but the language itself can be confusing, alienating and sometimes ambiguous. Traditionally doctors have used specialist terminology to demonstrate their scientific credentials and to provide clarity. Professional language also serves the additional purpose of creating a secret code which ordinary people can't understand. This puts doctors above and beyond the general population because it signals that they have complex and specialist knowledge. As midwifery became professionalised in the 20th century, midwives too took on professional language. This was partly to allow them to communicate on more equal terms with doctors but also to signal themselves as professionals with more knowledge and expertise than the women they cared for (Marsh, 2019). Over time some of this language has become clearer but there are still elements that are mysterious and even frightening to families.

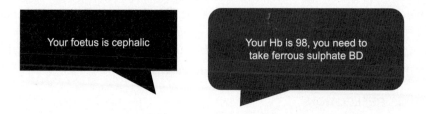

These phrases could be a source of confusion or anxiety to the people hearing them. The same applies to the notes we take. The following example is a simple record of an antenatal appointment.

| 09.11.22 | 36/40 | Long lie | Ceph/free | FH 136 FMF | | 110/72 | Urine NAD | CMW |

To a professional it will seem clear and helpful. To a pregnant person it could be confusing. Just because we understand things, never assume other people do—even other colleagues. Be clear in communication in all circumstances and don't be afraid to check understanding or meaning if it is something you are not clear about. As Marsh (2019) has pointed out, the use of medical jargon has implications for our ethical practice as well as being understood. It is hard for people to give informed consent, to be part of decision-making or to be at the centre of care if they don't understand what is being communicated.

## Conclusion

In this chapter we have explored what we mean by the idea of 'communication' in general and in midwifery practice. We considered what good and bad communication looks like and the impact that this might have on us, families and the service. Communication challenges have been put in their historical and sociological context and the professional and regulatory requirements around communication have been highlighted. The attributes of the midwife as professional friend have been discussed, as have barriers to communication in practice. The principles and expectations of effective communication are relevant to every chapter in this book and will be revisited in the context of each subject and issue.

## References

Boyd, C., & Sellers, L. (1982). *The British way of birth*. Pan Books.
CQC, (2021). *The duty of candour: guidance for providers*. Care Quality Commission. https://www.cqc.org.uk/sites/default/files/20210421%20The%20duty%20of%20candour%20-%20guidance%20for%20providers.pdf.
Expert Maternity Group, (1992). *Changing childbirth*. HMSO.
ICM. (2014). *International code of ethics for midwives*. https://www.internationalmidwives.org/our-work/policy-and-practice/icm-definitions.html
Marsh, A. (2019). The importance of language in maternity services. *British Journal of Midwifery*, *27*(5). https://www.britishjournalofmidwifery.com/content/other/the-importance-of-language-in-maternity-services.
McIntosh, T. (2012). *A social history of maternity care*. Routledge.
McIntosh, T. (2017). Changing messages about place of birth in *Mother and Baby* magazine between 1956 and 1992. *Midwifery*, *54*, 1–6.
National Maternity Review, (2016). *Better births: Improving outcomes of maternity services in England*. NHS England.
NMC. (2019). *Standards of proficiency for midwives*. https://www.nmc.org.uk/standards/standards-for-midwives/standards-of-proficiency-for-midwives/
Ockenden, D. (2022). *Ockenden report – final: Findings, conclusions and essential actions from the independent review of maternity services at The Shrewsbury and Telford Hospital NHS Trust*. Her Majesty's Stationery Office (HMSO). https://assets.publishing.service.gov.uk/government/uploads/system/uploads/attachment_data/file/1064302/Final-Ockenden-Report-web-accessible.pdf.
Pairman, S., Pincombe, J., Thorogood, C., & Tracy, S. K. (2006). *Midwifery: preparation for practice*. Elsevier.
Rosengren, K. R. (2000). *Communication: An introduction*. Sage.
Smith, J. (1997). *Labour days: Having a baby before the birth of the National Health Service*. Jay Publishing.
Walsh, D. (1999). An ethnographic study of women's experience of partnership caseload midwifery practice: The professional as a friend. *Midwifery*, *15*, 165–176.

## Resources

Baston, H., Hall, J., & Henley-Einion, A. (2017). *Midwifery essentials: Volume 1, basics*. Elsevier.
 *Chapter 2 is a good summary of communication in midwifery.*
Peanut. (n.d.). *The #RenamingRevolution*. https://www.peanut-app.io/blog/renaming-revolution-glossary
 *The UK regulatory body sets out clearly what knowledge skills and attributes are expected of midwives in relation to communication.*

This online resource has been developed by women in response to the judgemental and negative language often used in the medical and maternity services. It was developed after a service user in the United States posted a video on social media discussing how the use of the term 'geriatric mother' made her feel as a pregnant woman in her 30 s.

NMC. (2019). *Standards of proficiency for midwives.* https://www.nmc.org.uk/standards/standards-for-midwives/standards-of-proficiency-for-midwives/

# CHAPTER 4

# Theories of Communication and Counselling

Cathy Ashwin ■ Rebekah Wells

## Introduction

The ability to communicate effectively with women, their families, colleagues and associated health care professionals is an essential component of being a midwife. You may already consider that you are a good communicator—you can talk and hold a conversation with most people—what else is there to know? As we have seen in Chapter 3, to communicate means much more than just talking, and encompasses the giving, sharing and exchanging of information (Gopee, 2008). This chapter will explore some models of communication and consider how we might use them in midwifery practice. We will then look in detail at counselling skills as a particular type of communication that midwives use daily. To enable a counselling situation to achieve positive outcomes for all concerned, the midwife must have an excellent understanding of communicating. This chapter explores communication within a counselling situation and offers both theoretical and practical approaches. In so doing it offers a deeper understanding of the nuances of the midwife–woman relationship and the effect this may have on the long- or short-term outcomes. Finally, a further area that cannot be overlooked is the practice supervisor–student relationship, where again there is a need for excellent communication skills and on occasion the counselling skills that may be required to support the student through education and beyond into their professional career.

Communication can be linear, interactional or transactional depending on the situation, sometimes requiring a combination of these models. This will be discussed within the chapter. To enable a constructive relationship to develop between the midwife and the person involved in the situation, the midwife must have a high degree of self-awareness and be cognisant of their limitations. The aims of this chapter are to enhance the reader's knowledge of the power of communication and to encourage insight into how certain behaviours can enable or harm the recipient of the counselling situation. In considering the principles of counselling, the different forms of communication, including verbal/nonverbal, written and oral, will be included in the discussion.

## Models of Communication

The first section of this chapter looks briefly at models of communication. We begin by considering some of the building blocks of communication theory and then consider specific approaches that are useful in therapeutic or helping roles such as midwifery. It is not important to remember the details of theories but to appreciate that even subconsciously, we all use models and styles of communicating. Some have argued that communication is so subtle and nuanced, and so dependent on time and place, that it cannot be defined in general terms. However, Adami (2016) suggests communication can be seen broadly as a message conveyed through social interaction. Following this definition, we could argue that the aim of imparting information by communicating is to decrease uncertainty:

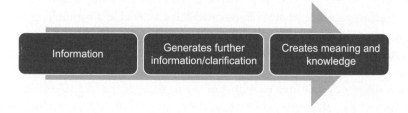

This is certainly what a lot of midwife–client interactions can look like—the midwife gives information which then leads to knowledge and understanding in the client. Of course, sometimes the information is misheard or misunderstood and at other times it might be seen as confusing or irrelevant. The idea of actively passing information to a passive recipient is important—but should only be a small element of our communication as midwives. Midwives enter the profession with communication skills acquired through previous experience and go on to develop and improve their skills throughout midwifery education, drawing on the expertise of their mentors, preceptors and colleagues. We all have our own experiences of communicating and ways of doing it. However, the skill of making effective, trusting relationships quickly, as in the first encounter between midwife and woman, is complex and demanding. It is a skill we learn over time as we practice and watch others. Often in our earliest days as students, our encounters are more taken up with giving information to women. We have learned the information and passing it on allows us to feel in control of the situation and to feel that we have done our job.

Over time, and as our knowledge and confidence grows, we tend to find that communication with women becomes less about handing over parcels of information and more about a structured conversation. The idea of a conversation is that it involves two active participants rather than one actively handing out information and the other passively receiving it. Women need this communication link with the midwife and should feel able to respond as well as listen to the information imparted, thus a two-way process is formed (Kirkham, 1993). This sits well with the transactional model of communication as described later. Pillay and Smith (2019) emphasise the importance of the relationship between woman and midwife, illustrating the dangers of poor communication resulting in a negative experience for the woman. Moreover, the safety of the woman and baby could be compromised if communication channels break down, specifically in interprofessional relationships—look at Chapter 8 to explore communication in complex cases where the breakdown of the relationship is a possibility and ways that this can be managed.

Midwives and women are both senders and receivers of communication; however, the interpretation of the messages conveyed can be affected by cultural differences, barriers to understanding, or even emotions such as anxiety or fear. We cannot always be sure that what we communicate is received as we intended. For this reason, it is vital that we always check understanding and interpretation—just because you have said something, it does not mean it has been heard, never mind understood as you intended. As we saw in Chapter 3, every time we communicate, we are saying something about our beliefs, expectations, culture and emotions. Midwifery is a diverse profession and midwives require the ability to communicate and counsel people on many different levels, which can be challenging at times, therefore it is useful to have a range of models and tools to fit individual situations.

### PRACTICE POINTS

Examples of potential barriers to communication:
- Not sharing a language
- Language processing challenges
- Emotions—e.g., fear, anxiety
- Not understanding cultural signifiers in language, expression and body language
- Basic needs not being met—e.g., feeling cold, hungry, tired, scared
- The use of complex scientific or technical jargon
- Busyness and lack of time

In recent times the COVID pandemic has made society think very differently about how to communicate, and midwifery is no exception, with the use of social media and online meeting facilities. These have been an alternative way of communicating during the period when meeting physically was not possible. This has been a positive innovation and has enabled midwives to maintain communication with the women they have been supporting through pregnancy and is likely to continue in some circumstances in the future. On balance, social media has been a help to many; nonetheless, vigilance must be maintained by midwives as some women may access inaccurate or inappropriate information and wellbeing is compromised (see Chapter 14 for a discussion on social media).

**QUICK REFLECTION**

Virtual meetings online have kept communication channels open between midwives and women during the recent pandemic 'lockdown'. What are the advantages and disadvantages of this method of communicating?

There are many models of communication, and these can be tailored to the situation requiring a particular way of communicating. The linear, interactional and transactional models can be adapted to many situations in the business world and in health care (Figs. 4.1–4.3). A further example is the RAV (recognising, acknowledging and validating) model which is suited to health care situations in both the service user–midwife scenarios as well as the practice supervisor–student relationship (Fig. 4.4). The RAV model can be integrated and used within a counselling session.

Kuznar and Yager (2020) discuss the history of communication models and suggest that the first linear model was attributed to Aristotle (ca 350 BCE). However, the most significant developments in communication modelling were developed in the periods encompassing the two world wars, where communication was vital in relaying information within the armed forces (see Fig. 4.1).

Sender.............message...............channel (could be telephone)...............receiver

**Fig. 4.1**   A linear model of communication.

Sender........message.....channel .....receiver.....feedback to sender

**Fig. 4.2**   An interactional model of communication.

| Encode | Context | Decode |
| Sender............Message............Receiver | | |
| Decode | Channel | Encode and sends feedback |

**Fig. 4.3**   A transactional model of communication.

## THE LINEAR MODEL

The linear model is a simple one-way system of relaying information from the person holding the information to be transmitted to the recipient and does not involve or require a response. The information may be given verbally face to face, by telephone, a written message or by email and is termed as an encoded message. It is then left to the receiver of the information to decode the message and act upon it as they consider appropriate, or they may decide to do nothing at all and either discard or store the information. Kuznar and Yager (2020) consider this model as a first step in communicating; however, important steps are missing to form meaningful two-way communication.

### EXAMPLE OF LINEAR COMMUNICATION

**Voice message left by a midwife on a woman's phone:** Your iron is lower than we would like. Could you please pop to the surgery and collect a prescription for ferrous sulphate—the instructions for taking it are on the packet.

*At first glance this looks like a clear message which transmits information (about iron levels) and an instruction (about collecting a prescription). However, it assumes that information about low iron will be understood. This information may cause confusion or anxiety. Alternatively, if it is not understood by the woman receiving the message it may be ignored. The midwife also assumes that 'ferrous sulphate' will be understood and related to low iron—but this is a specific professional term that might not be understood by the woman. Because the communication is linear—one-way—then the midwife cannot check understanding or even check that the woman is able to collect and take the prescription.*

## THE INTERACTIONAL MODEL

This model moves a step on from the linear model because it includes the possibility of a response to the initial message. The incoming message is received, and the recipient then considers the content and meaning which results in sending back a response. The response may be affected by the conditions in which the response was received, i.e. external environmental factors or internal dilemmas happening during this exchange of messages (see Fig. 4.2).

Although these models feel very formal and perhaps not relevant to real-world situations, they do in fact form the basis of the structured communication tools used in the maternity services. Tools for communicating at handover or escalating emergencies such as SBAR (**S**ituation–**B**ackground–**A**ssessment–**R**ecommendation) are examples of linear/interactional communication. Information is packaged and passed on in a particular format to make it easy to understand. Sometimes it is responded to or communicated on in an equally structured way. The idea behind tools such as SBAR is to ensure clarity and meaning, so important issues are not missed or misunderstood. Chapter 13 explores how tools such as SBAR can be used in challenging situations to minimise communication breakdown between professionals.

## THE TRANSACTIONAL MODEL

In an ideal world the transactional model would be suited to many situations as it allows the exchange of information, ideas and messages to be conveyed between the originator of the first message and the receiver of the information. In this situation both parties are involved in the exchange of messages and can respond accordingly. Each involved individual can both impart information and consider the implications of such information. Ideally any information which is unclear, ambiguous or inappropriate can be questioned and clarified to avoid misinterpretation (see Fig. 4.3).

This model forms the basis for many of the conversations we have with women and families. In that initial encounter we may give information, but the woman responds with questions and information of her own. In this way a relationship, and a shared understanding, begins to build.

### EXAMPLE OF TRANSACTIONAL COMMUNICATION

*Midwife*: Of course, you know that breastfeeding is recommended for the first 6 months, but the choice is entirely yours.
*Woman*: I tried to breastfeed last time but really struggled. I'd like to try again—will there be help available?
*Midwife*: Absolutely—we now have two infant feeding specialist midwives. I will put you in touch with them. There is also a local breastfeeding peer support group.
*Woman*: I'm not keen on groups—they make me anxious. But the specialist support sounds good.
  *In this example the midwife relays information about feeding. The woman responds—making this a conversation. By the end of this brief encounter the woman has more of a sense of the support available to her and the midwife begins to understand the woman better as an individual.*

## RECOGNISING, ACKNOWLEDGING AND VALIDATING: THE RAV MODEL

There are certain conditions that are essential in developing a therapeutic relationship with a person experiencing a difficult, unusual or different situation and these comprise *recognising, acknowledging* and *validating* (RAV) the concerns of the individual involved. The RAV model can be used in everyday situations, for example with friends and family as well as professional encounters. For example, if a friend has been to the hair salon but is not happy with her new style, RAV can be used to respond to their emotions and concerns. However, RAV lends itself particularly well to counselling situations where the need to gain the confidence of the person requiring help is paramount in building a trusting relationship.

The first step in the relationship is **R**ecognising there is a situation and eliciting the appropriate genuine responses, demonstrating empathy using verbal and nonverbal cues. **A**cknowledging the problem is the next step in the RAV model; building up a rapport with the person concerned will contribute to the therapeutic relationship forming. Finally, **V**alidating the problem is important in demonstrating that the person's concerns are real and not trivial. At this stage, the midwife building up the relationship with the person in need of help should ask questions to elicit more information. By doing so we further validate the issues requiring investigation. RAV will help clarify the situation and begin to build the relationship; this may be all the recipient needs at this stage. If the problem requires deeper discussion, then RAV will provide the building blocks to move into a more formalised counselling session.

Prior to undertaking any counselling, it is the midwife's responsibility to take ethical considerations into account. Where counselling skills may be applied in any practice or personal situation, formal counselling should only take place if the midwife is trained and competent to undertake this role—counselling sessions should always be beneficial to the person receiving counselling and never harmful. Offering or providing counselling to a woman in a situation beyond the competency of the midwife/counsellor would be unethical and dangerous. Careful consideration must be given before offering counselling support to ensure it will be of help (beneficence) and not cause harm (maleficence). Therefore, building a therapeutic relationship with someone having a difficult experience requires competence and confidence in the required skills of communication and counselling, an open positive attitude and self-awareness of one's own limitations.

As we saw in Chapter 3, communication begins at birth through eye contact, touch and sound, developing into verbal communication for most people. However, communicating with others in a counselling situation takes practice and involves learning new skills or honing those we already have. Initially we are unaware of what we do not know and thus incompetent, moving through to being aware of our lack of skills but still unable to achieve this state. As our skills develop, we are not always aware of using them until finally we are. As a midwife we should be comfortable in developing and using basic counselling skills, although we are not counsellors. In all cases it is important to act only within our scope of practice and to refer on when situations are beyond our remit and expertise.

## What Is Counselling?

At its core, counselling is simply communicating through constructive and purposeful dialogue in such a way that one person, experiencing a problem, can be helped by another. The role of the counsellor is to facilitate the individual in identifying the problem and then working with them to seek out practical solutions. In essence, the aim of counselling is to give comfort to the person in need while aiding them to gain insight into their concern. This in turn can generate self-awareness and will ultimately support the individual in being able to move forward with confidence.

While not all midwives will be trained counsellors, all can apply counselling principles in their practice. It is important to offer care that remains within the scope of personal practice, and effective signposting and referring on are key skills for midwives. However, basic counselling skills employed by a midwife will contribute to positive experiences throughout the childbearing year. In midwifery most counselling situations will be one-to one between the midwife and the pregnant or postnatal client. On occasion it may involve couples, and less commonly it could involve a small group, for example, where a surrogate is also involved. These instances may be challenging and where possible would ideally be undertaken by those more confident in the skills of counselling.

The process of counselling in a midwifery context may often comprise only a single meeting, whereas for those offering specific counselling services, including within the maternity service, it could involve a long-term ongoing relationship. This may depend upon whether the concern is an immediate crisis or an incremental development. Each scenario will be unique and may call for specific counselling skills, but in the moment within the practice setting the overriding requirement is that the relationship between the woman and midwife is a solid healthy base from which to start.

## BASIC COUNSELLING SKILLS

To enable constructive counselling to take place certain conditions need to be met, core skills need to be utilised and key principles need to be applied.

| Core Skills | Key Principles |
| --- | --- |
| Listening | Listening rather than talking |
| Demonstrating empathy | Being empathic rather than dismissive |
| Being nonjudgemental | Accepting rather than judging |
| Being genuine and real | Looking for goals rather than solutions |

(Nelson-Jones, 2012)

These three main core attitudinal conditions of **empathy, unconditional positive regard** and **genuineness** (sometimes referred to as congruence) are mentioned frequently in counselling texts but often it is assumed that we understand what these words really mean and how it makes a person feel. **Empathy** is seeing things through the client's eyes and trying to understand things from their perspective. This is quite different from sympathy, where we still see things from our own perspective and can be portrayed more as pity. In practice, empathy can often be applied through conversation by confirming with the client how they feel about a situation, rather than expressing sympathy, as this avoids implying how you would feel in the situation.

Demonstrating **unconditional positive regard** sounds complex but is actually the simplest of the core conditions. It means accepting the client as they are and taking a nonjudgemental approach to them and to what they say. To do this, we must suspend our personal beliefs and values. This is what we do every day as professionals; we 'park' our own feeling and beliefs in order to give the most appropriate support to those in our care.

**Genuineness** is an authentic commitment to support the client, and to build the working relationship with them, supporting them as they explore positive changes (Egan, 1986). In practice this may be expressed by showing a genuine interest in the client, remembering details they have shared with you and remaining continually engaged. Genuineness, or a lack thereof, is normally transparent to the client and therefore it is vital to express this honestly.

Beyond the triad of unconditional positive regard, empathy and genuineness there are several other key communication skills involved in counselling.

- Active listening—that is listening fully to actually hear the meaning of what is being expressed. Active listening includes conversation that is not only words, but the way in which the words are used and aspects of body language as well.
- Questioning—that is both open ended to aid the client in exploring thoughts or feelings and closed ended to define the narrative or to elicit information.
- Paraphrasing—that is the capacity to concisely and accurately reiterate and clarify the main sentiments of what a client has expressed.
- Reflecting—that is the ability to allow a client to see themselves and their own feelings more clearly by reflecting back to them what they have expressed.
- Summarising—that is drawing together key points and highlighting future directions.
- Challenging—that is the process of reassessing the narrative. This is an advanced counselling skill, but in practice involves the counsellor challenging the client to really assess the narrative of their story and to fully and critically consider the details.

The application of these key skills will be influenced to a certain extent by the setting in which the counselling is taking place. It is therefore important to take this into consideration when embarking on a counselling session. The situation may be impromptu and happen at the side of the bed in a hospital setting, it could be in the client's home, or it may be a prearranged appointment in a designated office. In all situations, where possible, the SOLER acronym should be considered and implemented.

**S**—face squarely (implying 'I am with you')

**O**—open posture (nonthreatening, genuine)

**L**—lean forward (showing interest, ready to listen)

**E**—make eye contact (again showing interest, avoid eye rolling or staring intently)

**R**—relax (this will help the client to feel more comfortable and willing to communicate)

---

**COFFEE BREAK ACTIVITY**

Consider how it would feel to be in a counselling situation where you are the person with the concern. Starting with this list, think about the qualities you would expect, or want, from the person helping you. Can you add to this list?
- Empathy
- Warmth
- Honesty
- Unbiased
- Respectful
- Confidential
- Attentive
- Understandable
- Authority
- Transparency—to be aware of their own emotional issues

---

Not everything can be solved by counselling alone—sometimes a more practical solution may be required instead or as well—therefore it is essential to first identify what the situation is. Equally, there will be times when a midwife would consider a counselling approach where the client would not see the need, and vice versa. This highlights the need to individualise the approach when applying counselling skills in practice.

---

**PRACTICE POINTS**

Giving information such as the result of a screening test.

This is *news* to the woman and a neutral tone is essential when giving this information. News is neither good nor bad, rather its identity is determined by how it is interpreted by the recipient. What one person may perceive as 'bad' news may be received positively by another.

---

When applying counselling skills, first the problem needs to be identified. This can then be followed by understanding the impact it is having on the individual. In the professional context it is important not to give personal advice but to draw on unbiased evidence-based information which can later guide the client's decision-making. Consider how the information is being received and if there are any external forces which may be affecting the individual's thought processes. Carefully consider and discuss what you can help with and any areas that may block this journey.

**Case Study**

Rachel, age 33, office manager in a high-profile company.
 Partner, Jo, age 30, works in hospitality industry.
 Rachel and Jo have been together for 10 years and are a very close couple. The couple live a very 'organised' life and plan everything they do, including this first pregnancy. They attended all the antenatal appointments, had relevant blood tests and joined groups to prepare for the birth. The pregnancy progressed uneventfully but Rachel became a little anxious that she was unable to know the exact date the baby would be born. However, after discussion Rachel and Jo opted to have a Caesarean section. This pleased the couple as it suited their need to be organised. A week before the date planned for the birth Rachel went into spontaneous labour and gave birth vaginally after only 3 hours from the start of contractions. The baby boy looked healthy at birth, cried spontaneously and breastfed well. On examination concerns were raised by the midwife caring for Rachel and the baby and subsequent consultations revealed the baby had Trisomy 21.
 Rachel and Jo were in extreme shock as this situation did not fit with their organised lives and expectations.
• As the midwife how would you feel and react to this information?
• How would you approach the parents? (Consider verbal and visual communication.)
• Would you feel competent in progressing the communication to a counselling situation when appropriate?
• Where would you get support?

## COUNSELLING MODELS

There are many different types of counselling, each relevant dependent on the circumstance. Although some of these are for specific situations, the main tenets of counselling principles still apply and indeed several if not all can be used in midwifery settings, either singly or combined. Not all the models can be discussed within this chapter so an overview will be given of some of the main ones which may be most useful.

### The Person-Centred Approach

The person-centred (humanistic) approach developed by Carl Rogers in the 1940s–1950s is one of the early and more recognised forms of counselling. This approach is useful when supporting others with a problem, particularly within midwifery, where the midwife has the knowledge to help that person. Good communication skills are essential in all counselling situations and models but may be more relatable in the person-centred approach—often the person needing help may not be seeking a solution to a definitive problem but may purely need someone to talk to. This can be ideal in such scenarios as a conversation develops organically and ideas are formed. Feminist counselling also fits well with the person-centred approach and midwifery as it does not always seek to find answers but allows the person to open to ideas. Chaplin (1999) considers that in life we move through

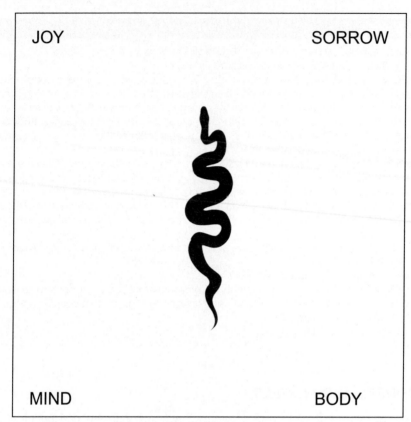

**Fig. 4.4**   Models of feminist counselling—the rhythm model.

inner difficult journeys fraught with hazards and that counselling is about making journeys through these conditions. Fig. 4.4 illustrates the rhythm of life, weaving in and out like a snake moving through times of joy and sorrow, the mind and the body. During this rhythm therapeutic changes can take place with counselling. Furthermore, Rogers (1980) believed that when the counsellor had the appropriate skills to counsel then a therapeutic change could take place. In addition, Rogers (1980) suggests the 'client' has deep knowledge of their own resources for moving forward and can also then help themselves. To enable this therapy to happen two people must be in contact and be in different places at this point; that is, the person requiring support will be in a state of incongruence, vulnerable and anxious. The person giving the support, the 'counsellor', will be congruent in the relationship. The counsellor will experience unconditional positive regard for the person requiring help, also experiencing and being able to demonstrate an empathic understanding of their internal set of beliefs that determines their behaviours. Respect, genuineness, empathy and warmth are all qualities which the counsellor should demonstrate when with the client, giving confidence with the aim to empower them to work through their issues and concerns.

Although the counsellor is the person leading the counselling therapy, it is important to stress that they are not the expert but are working together with the client towards an equal relationship. The counsellor must be aware of where the client is on their stage of the journey and be able to adapt to be congruent with their thoughts and feelings. In essence, this approach considers that human nature is inherently a constructive way of being as opposed to destructive. Furthermore, it is human nature to be social and as such, self-regard is a basic need (Maslow, 1943).

## The Skilled Helper

Counselling can occasionally be a situation where the person encountering a problem may only wish for the concern to be validated and for someone to listen to them; however, more constructive support is required. In the 'skilled helper' model (Egan & Reese, 2021) the person in need of help is supported in working through the problem and deciding on action. As with all counselling situations Egan and Reese (2021) recommend a quiet confidential environment, enabling open non-judgemental communication. The helper (counsellor) encourages the person being counselled to think more deeply about their concerns and themselves with the aim to develop ways to manage the problem and move on. This is facilitated through three stages:

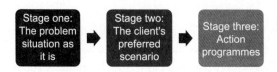

These stages give a logical plan, flowing through the problem and resulting in a solution the person can work with. For this to have a successful outcome, both the counsellor (midwife) and the client (pregnant/postnatal client or student midwife) must always be aware of which stage they are at. It would be very easy to use this as a 'quick fix', where the counsellor 'tells' the client what to do and does not work through the stages together. This model works well in practice between a student and their preceptor as it lends itself well to practical problems that may arise, such as professional relationships (see Case Study).

## Case Study

Leonie is a first-year student entering midwifery almost straight from school. She is friendly, eager to please and learn. The people she cares for under supervision like to talk to her and often ask questions she is unable to answer—Leonie tries to answer them as she is a little in awe of her supervisor and anxious not to appear unknowledgeable. However, Leonie's supervisor was not very positive when they had a mid-placement meeting. Leonie was quite taken aback and upset as this was not the response she had been expecting and became quite withdrawn and reluctant to engage with the women.

The tutor noticed Leonie was also quiet in lectures and reluctant to join in discussions. On further investigation Leonie opened up to the lecturer about her concerns with her supervisor. The lecturer used the 'skilled helper model' to support Leonie through her negative experiences.

They discussed the problem and concluded there were difficulties between Leonie and her supervisor. It was agreed to hold a tripartite meeting to discuss the issues. It transpired that Leonie was very keen to achieve but felt afraid of the supervisor as she had not had a very welcoming start on the placement, so gave advice to the women based on her pregnant sisters' experience. The supervisor had not had much experience with younger students and misinterpreted Leonie's enthusiasm as 'a cocky student'. The tutor discussed what Leonie wanted to do to help resolve the situation, then they all worked out an action plan to make this happen.

Consider:
- How does this scenario make you feel?
- What would you do as Leonie, the supervisor and the tutor?
- Was this appropriate to speak to the tutor in the first instance?
- Who else could Leonie speak to?
- Is there anything you would have done differently?
- What communication signals may have been evident to make the assumption that Leonie was 'cocky' and that the supervisor was unhelpful to Leonie?

## The Six Category Intervention

Heron first developed the 'Six Category Intervention', which is loosely divided into two areas—authoritative and facilitative (Heron, 2001). It is under these two headings that the six categories reside (see Fig. 4.5.). This model of counselling is suitable for use in midwifery, but careful consideration must be given to the situations it is used in as it could be harmful if used in inappropriate situations.

Three categories—prescriptive, informative and confronting—are used authoritatively, which may appear counterintuitive to the previous models which advocate the person counselled to be the one to find the solutions to the problem. However, in certain situations this would be appropriate. For example, at the first booking appointment when people may be seeking information on screening tests, the midwife would be taking a more informative stance. Alternatively, a midwife on a home visit may observe someone in the house behaving inappropriately, such as smoking around the baby, and here confronting communication and counselling would take place.

When examining the facilitative side of the interventions, the midwife/counsellor is enabling the client to have greater autonomy and responsibility around the

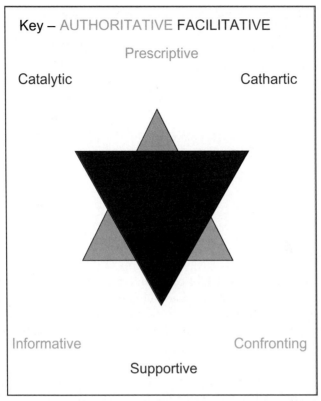

**Fig. 4.5**  Heron's six categories of counselling intervention. From Heron, J. (2001). *Helping the client. A creative practical guide* (5th ed.). Sage Publications Ltd.

situation, affirming worth and positivity. For example, the woman may be struggling with breastfeeding, so before an action plan can be made the midwife/counsellor facilitates the woman to express her emotions, which can be cathartic, enabling her to move on (catalytic stage) to then provide support going forward.

There are potential stumbling blocks with this model in the context of midwifery. First, the midwife (counsellor) may misunderstand the problem and go off in another direction, leaving the woman confused and unsure of what is expected. Secondly, the midwife may also take an unhealthy interest in the problem and 'dig too deep' into the issue, seeking inappropriate or unhelpful information. Thirdly, the woman may misinterpret the midwife and assume they will find a solution to the problem for them. This again highlights the importance of carefully applying counselling skills to each unique situation.

### Case Study

Lucy, aged 27, attends an antenatal clinic. This is her third pregnancy but she has miscarried the first two babies. The midwife has not met Lucy before and has not read her history (Lucy has diabetes and has been a victim of domestic abuse in the past with a different partner). Lucy appears in a rush and excitable and the midwife thought she could detect a smell of alcohol around her. She was accompanied by her new partner who seemed very attentive.

Consider:
- What do you think this scenario portraying?
- Are you making assumptions?
- As the midwife, how would you approach the couple?
- Using Heron's six category Intervention, discuss with a colleague the steps you would take to understand and help Lucy.

## Conclusion

This chapter has explored models of communication and counselling with the aim of deepening understanding of the value and importance of the art of communication in midwifery. As mentioned at the start of the chapter, we may think we are all good communicators, but have we really considered the impact on others when utilising other skills besides verbal? The nonverbal ways we communicate can have a much greater impact than speech alone.

Midwives are in a privileged position to offer support throughout pregnancy, birth and the postnatal period, especially in difficult circumstances. This can be enhanced by having greater self-awareness of our communication skills, and our less positive verbal and nonverbal skills. Counselling is a significant area of midwifery practice and as such we must strive to support those faced with difficult news to the best of our abilities. This includes recognising when a situation is beyond our competency and being able to signpost to the appropriate help. The examples of counselling models within this chapter are well tried and tested methods and are suited to most midwifery situations but are by no means the only ones in use today.

The most valuable message to take from this chapter is to always be honest, genuine and empathic in your interactions. Consider how your communication is received and interpreted by the people you speak to and how you would feel if on the receiving end of your help.

### EXERCISES IN COMMUNICATION

These exercises are best undertaken in groups of three so one person can provide feedback as an observer. Each exercise should only last around 5 minutes. Then discuss how each exercise makes you feel and how it can be corrected.
1. One person stays silent and shows no facial expression. The other person tries to talk to them about a problem they have.

2. One person talks about their problem again and the 'listener' fidgets, looks at their phone, sighs and makes inappropriate facial expressions.
3. The listener has their back to the person while they talk.
4. This time while the story/problem is being told the second person/listener keeps interrupting and comparing the problem with their own life.
5. Consider how both of you are sitting (SOLER). This time the person listening is attentive and listens to the story being told and makes appropriate eye contact and comments. How different does this feel and what else if anything can you do to improve this situation?

## References

Adami, C. (2016). What is information? *Philosophical Transactions. Series A, Mathematical, Physical, and Engineering Sciences, 374*(2063), 20150230. https://doi.org/10.1098/rsta.2015.0230.

Chaplin, J. (1999). *Feminist counselling in action* (2nd ed.). Sage Publications Ltd.

Egan, G. (1986). *The skilled helper: A systematic approach to effective helping.* Brooks/Cole Publishing Company.

Egan, G., & Reese, R. (2021). *The skilled helper* (3rd ed.). Cengage Learning EMEA.

Gopee, N. (2008). *Mentoring and supervision in healthcare.* Sage Publications Ltd.

Heron, J. (2001). *Helping the client. A creative practical guide* (5th ed.). Sage Publications Ltd.

Kirkham, M. (1993). Communication in midwifery. In J. Alexander, V. Levy, & S. Roch (Eds.), *Midwifery practice* (pp. 1–19). Palgrave.

Kuznar, L. A., & Yager, M. (2020). The development of communication models. *Prepared for: Strategic Multilayer Assessment Integrating Information in Joint Operations (IIJO)*, 1–9. NSI.

Maslow, A. H. (1943). A theory of human motivation. *Psychological Review, 50*(4), 370–396.

Nelson-Jones, R. (2012). *Introduction to counselling skills* (4th ed.). Sage Publications Ltd.

Pillay, L., & Smith, L. (2019). Communicating effectivelyin midwifery education and practice. Chapter 3. In J. E. Marshall (Ed.), *Myles professional studies for midwifery education* (pp. 37–54). Elsevier.

Rogers, C. R. (1980). *A way of being.* Houghton Mifflin.

## Resources

British Association for Counselling and Psychotherapy (BACP). https://www.bacp.co.uk/
   *The British Association for Counselling and Psychotherapy is the professional association for members of the counselling professions in the UK. The website has resources, links and useful information.*

Consultations 4 Health. (2019). *The RAV model.* University of East Anglia (UEA) Norwich Medical School. https://www.youtube.com/@Consultations4Health
   *Consultations 4 Health have produced a range of videos about communication with patients/clients in a range of health situations. The videos include this one on the RAV model, and others on active listening, building a rapport and inclusive language.*

# CHAPTER 5

# Communicating Ideas

Tania Staras

## Introduction

As previous chapters have already demonstrated, communication is key to midwifery care. Despite being very much a hands-on physical job, it is communication which allows us to build relationships with families and to plan care and to provide advocacy, support and compassion when required. Midwives communicate with their voices, their hands, their eyes and their bodies. The service communicates through room layouts, signage, uniforms and attitudes. Everything we do is communication and drives the professional care that we provide.

At the heart of this is the childbearing woman or person. In many ways pregnancy, labour, birth and the postnatal period—the human communication which goes with them—stand outside time. People giving birth in ancient Rome, Victorian London or modern China would recognise each other's experiences. The physiological process of parturition has strong elements of constancy. As a result of this, the idea of communication in the childbearing year seems superficially to be uncomplicated. Whether in ancient Rome, Victorian London or modern China, kindness and care are needed. However, this is just the first layer of the process. The society that we live in and our culture, beliefs and expectations all play a part in how we view pregnancy and birth. This means that the biological process becomes wrapped in wider concerns, and communication must reflect these. If we put ancient Rome or Victorian London to one side and concentrate on contemporary societies, there are a variety of issues that have an impact on how pregnancy and birth are thought about, managed and communicated.

### COFFEE BREAK ACTIVITY

- Which of the issues in Fig. 5.1 do you think is the most important to communicate when giving care?
- Which do you think is the most difficult to communicate to families?

Fig. 5.1 demonstrates a selection of social and cultural issues which are 'attached' to pregnancy and birth in the modern world. The list is not exhaustive but highlights

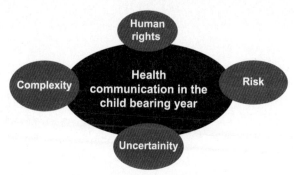

**Fig. 5.1**  Issues related to health communication and childbirth.

the complexity of providing responsive professional care. This chapter works through the elements in the diagram to explore the practicalities of communicating ideas. It considers the challenges of doing this in a way that is clear and responsive but also accepts ambiguity. The chapter critically considers how midwives understand and articulate ideas such as risk and uncertainty.

We begin with a brief exploration of **health communication** and why it matters to midwives and other caregivers. The chapter then explores the issues of **risk** and of **human rights** as they relate to the childbearing year and explains why we need to understand these ideas to be able to communicate safely, effectively and respectfully. We then consider how we can communicate **complexity** and **uncertainty** to families and look critically at the strategies midwives use to explain or manage tricky issues. Finally, we take a brief look at **moral issues** and communication within the maternity services and consider to what extent we communicate ethically and honestly, even when we think we are doing the right thing.

## Health Communication

Communication is at the centre of every aspect of our lives, from relationships to transactions to the work that we do. Every day we communicate with a wide variety of people, from friends and colleagues to children, other workers and, in maternity care, with clients and families. 'Health communication' describes the specific communication we do around the role as caregiver. The conversations that we have and information that we give might have general elements but are primarily targeted around communication about health and care. Cross et al. (2017) define health communication as an integral part of health promotion, and a lot of the research and discussion around health communication focuses on its role in health promotion and encouraging behaviour change. In midwifery we can clearly see this in conversations we might have about healthy eating or smoking cessation. These conversations are specific and targeted and designed with the goal of improved health in mind. The chapter on health promotion in this book explores in more detail how we can conduct these conversations in a meaningful and positive way which includes the client, rather than just leaving them feeling talked at.

**QUICK REFLECTION**
- What aspects of day-to-day communication with families do you find most challenging?
- Why do you think this is?

However, the idea of health communication is broader than just health promotion. It encompasses all the conversations we have with service users and families and all the information we share. Although it is a two-way process and involves listening, health communication is often seen as how we transmit specific and sometimes technical information. An example of this is work done in the South Africa by Sarangi and Gilstad (2014), which explored how midwife sonographers communicated to women and families what they were seeing on the ultrasound scan. As they point out, the machine became almost a participant in the conversation because both midwife and families directed their attention to it. The way that the conversation was structured also demonstrates features of the 'complexity' bubble we saw in Fig. 5.1 because it included both clinical and social aspects. Ultrasound screening has a medical surveillance role in that it can help to identify potential foetal abnormalities as well as assess foetal age, size, position and number. However, scanning has a powerful social role in modern society, with families using the experience to 'meet' their babies. At the same time families may also be seeking reassurance that their baby is healthy. Conversations around scanning are therefore multifaceted because they encompass all of these elements as well the uncertainty element of Fig. 5.1, because the scan cannot say for definite whether everything is normal and going to remain so.

To manage these conversations, Sarangi and Gilstad describe caregivers as using 'online' and 'offline' commentary. In online commentary they are talking directly about what is seen on screen, often not looking at the family and not expecting a response from them. In offline commentary they discuss and explain what they have seen and what it means directly with the family. The online commentary is medically focused whereas the offline commentary is much more social and includes reassurance.

Scanning is one example where health communication—that is communication between caregiver and care receiver—is made more complex by the presence of machinery in the room. This machinery—in this case the scanning equipment—becomes part of the conversation as the midwife and families both refer to it and include it in conversation. Another clear example of this in hospital-based care is the presence of the cardiotocography (CTG) machine. When women are labouring and a CTG machine is in use, this can become the focus of attention and conversation. Look at the following example of a conversation around CTG monitoring:

## Case Study

Midwife, student midwife, labouring woman and partner in the room. The foetal heart rate and contractions are being monitored via transducers strapped to the woman's abdomen. The results can be seen on the monitor screen.

*Student midwife:* The heart rate keeps disappearing.

*Woman:* Is everything ok?

*Midwife:* Everything is fine—it's just the machine that's playing up [to student] try adjusting it.

*Student midwife:* I think this is it now—its reading 150.

*Midwife:* What else can you tell me?

*Student midwife:* Baseline 130, variability of 10, no decelerations, acceleration to 150.

*Midwife* [to woman and partner]: That means that your little one is awake and happy.

**ACTIVITY**

- Think about 'online' and 'offline' communication; which aspects of this conversation do you think are online and which are offline?
- Which phrases are medical and which phrases are social? Why are different phrases used—does it depend on who is speaking, or who they are speaking to?
- If you were the woman and partner in this scenario, how might you feel?
- If you were the student, is there anything you would do differently?

As this activity reminds us, health communication is quite complicated because it is trying to do a lot of different things at once, including educating, reassuring, surveying and checking. We flip between technical and everyday language but need to bear in mind how it is received and understood by all the people in the room. In practice it is vital to be clear about what we are communicating, who our audience is and what the purpose of our communication is.

Of course, there are many aspects of care which require juggling between different types of communication, as in the earlier example, but where the information being conveyed is not necessarily complex or challenging. However, there are many other aspects of care where health communication plays a vital role in explaining complicated ideas or reaching decisions when there is no obvious right or wrong. One of these is induction of labour (IOL) in the absence of clear medical complications. The majority of IOLs in the UK occur to reduce the risk of foetal morbidity and mortality associated with prolonged pregnancy. We will look at the concept of 'risk' in more detail in the next section of this chapter, but as far as health communication is concerned, the challenge is to have clear conversations about choices around IOL and around the potential benefits and challenges of different approaches. Service users often report that information giving around the process and timeline of induction is vague, meaning that they may go into the process not understanding what it will entail, how long it will take, or what the chances of operative or instrumental deliveries are. They may feel that although they were notionally given a choice as to whether to proceed with IOL or not, in practice this didn't feel much like a choice. Similarly, midwives may feel constrained by their own understandings of the risks of prolonged pregnancy versus induction. For both families and caregivers, their personal belief systems and experiences form part of the background to the conversation—even if this is not always acknowledged. Equally, the way that the conversation is framed, whether emphasising the positive or negative aspects of the induction process, will make a difference to decision-making (Cheyne et al., 2012). In situations like this there is a trade-off between the risks and benefits of action, and the decision is not obvious or clear-cut. As caregivers we cannot change our philosophies or beliefs about care, but we should be aware of them and how they might impact on how we have conversations with families, the type of language we use and the way we frame discussions. We also need to be aware about how service users and families receive and process information and conversations to understand what they are hearing from us and what they are basing decisions on.

**PRACTICE POINTS**

- Health communication has a *clinical* and *social* aspect which includes education and reassurance.
- We transmit technical and complex information—to do this effectively we need to think about our audience and tailor our messages.
- We need to be aware that families will hear technical information we are sharing with other members of the care team.
- We need to think about how we interpret and explain this technical information.
- We need to be aware that our beliefs and understanding will affect how we will frame conversations with families.

The following sections explore the key issues highlighted in Fig. 5.1—risk, human rights, complexity and uncertainty—and relates them to health communication in the childbearing year.

# Risk

We have already briefly considered risk in relation to information giving around nonemergency IOL. Our ability to communicate risk depends on our understanding of the idea of risk in general and our beliefs about how it relates to the specific health issue we are discussing. Midwives have become used to using the language of risk over the last 30 years and reducing risk is seen as a basic function of any maternity care system. There are many writers who have tried to define risk in the context of modern maternity care (Coxon et al., 2012; Smith et al., 2012). In its original sense 'risk' is a statistical statement around the *likelihood* or *chance* of a given event occurring. It does not include a judgement about whether the event is positive or negative. However, in contemporary society 'risk' has become associated with a negative outcome, not just in the maternity services but in all areas of life. The national maternity review (NHS England, 2016), which came on the heels of critical reports about maternity care in England (particularly the Kirkup Report), argued that 'safety' should be at the centre of policy. In this context safety is seen as the opposite of risk—we maximise safety by minimising risk. Although we rarely put it in such stark terms, the end point of a failure to manage risk is serious injury or death.

**COFFEE BREAK ACTIVITY**

- What does the word 'risk' mean to you?
- Jot down three things that come to mind when you think about 'risk'.

Risk is not only about judgements of *obstetric* risk; it also includes wider issues such as social and organisational risk. Social risk might encompass maternal deprivation, refugee and non-English-speaking status (both significant risk factors for maternal mortality), or a lack of family or social support. Organisational risk includes relationships between different professional groups, and microfactors such as handovers and staffing levels and clinical rotation.

Decision-making to minimise risk might have a positive effect on one element of care and a negative effect on another. Consider the use of Caesarean section. As with IOL, there are times when a section is an unambiguous lifesaving procedure—in the case of placental abruption for example—and other situations when the decision about how to proceed is not so clear-cut. In these cases we need to communicate effectively with families so that people do not feel unconsciously manipulated into a particular course of action. Caesarean birth is carried out to reduce risks believed to be associated with vaginal birth in certain circumstances (e.g., breech presentation) but carries its own risks (major abdominal surgery). The risk of vaginal breech birth is to the baby; the solution of operative delivery transfers the majority of risk to the mother. This suggests that not all risks are equally discussed or carry equal weight; the risk to the foetus is often presented as more significant than the risk to the pregnant body. Seeking to minimise one risk through intervention may set off a chain of events—in this case the risks of Caesarean section for the mother may include:

- Physical recovery time from birth
- Possible infection
- Impact of losing planned and expected birth experience
- Impact on confidence and mental health
- Impact on next pregnancy/birth.

These things are harder to measure than the fact of a living baby and are therefore harder to discuss with families. However, we need to be careful about how we have these discussions, because we need to be honest and we need to be open about the fact that risk can never be completely eliminated. For most people risk equals fear and talking about risk in stark terms has the potential to be a tool of coercion and oppression. The language of maternity care may include choice and control for service users, but the centrality of the risk discourse trumps all these ideas and therefore the way we communicate notions of risk is really important.

How we talk about risk matters, but we also need to be aware that how people hear it and act on it will vary between individuals (Waters et al., 2014). People have different ideas about risk and what it means to them. They will also understand discussion of risk in different ways. Taking screening discussions as an example, caregivers tend to discuss the possibility of foetal abnormality in terms of ratios. So, we might say that a foetus has a 1:20 or 1:800 chance of having a particular condition. We cannot be sure that women and families will understand what ratios mean—and even if they do, we cannot assume that they will take the same view that we do or that another woman or family might. For example, one service user might see a risk of 1:200 as low and unproblematic whereas another might see it as very high and a source of great anxiety and distress. Therefore when we communicate any issue of chance, we need to remember that people do not interpret it rationally; emotions and experience, culture, spirituality and belief all play a part.

Pregnancy can make discussion of risk or probability even more complex because unlike health promotion activities, for example, which just involve one person ('if you continue to smoke you have a *risk* of developing lung cancer'), pregnancy risks might have an impact on at least two individuals—the pregnant person and the foetus. This might make people more risk averse than if they were just considering themselves and needs to be factored into discussion.

## PRACTICE POINTS

- Explore replacing the word 'risk' when we give care and talk to families.
- Using a thesaurus to explore the word 'risk' brings up a set of words associated with danger such as 'menace', 'threat', 'peril' and 'hazard'. These words are clearly very negative and potentially frightening. It also offers the opposite of 'risk' as 'safety'.
- Another set of words that can be used to replace 'risk' play on its original meaning of 'chance'. These words, which include 'possibility', 'likelihood' and 'chance' itself, are much less negative of ways of communicating.
- Every time you hear the word 'risk' being used to talk to families or see it written down, imagine it replaced with the word 'chance'. Try using 'chance' or 'possibility' when you are communicating with families and notice how it changes the tone of the discussion.
- Don't assume that people hear 'risk' or 'chance' in the same way that you mean it—check understanding.

# Human Rights

Giving care to women and families across the childbearing year has always been a deeply intimate and personal role. For most of history midwives were carers very much on a level with their clients; they learned their craft by doing and were not set apart in terms of education or social status. The language of human rights was implicit in the care given, not least because service users paid for attendance by doctors or midwives and therefore exerted a level of power within the relationship. Over the last century as pregnancy and birth have become more medicalised and more subject to expert control and surveillance, the relative position of families and caregivers has changed. The system now takes precedence and experts use their knowledge and training to manage the environment and process of pregnancy and birth.

Much of the effort in maternity care has revolved around making maternity care more accessible and safer for women and babies globally. However there has been increasing criticism of maternity systems which prioritise efficiency over care and compassion, and it is realised that good care is about more than physical safety. Good care is that which promotes wellbeing and psychological health and puts the person receiving care at the centre rather than just seeing them as part of a system (Lokugamage & Pathberiya, 2017). The language of human rights is increasingly used in maternity care to explore broad issues of care. The concept of human rights covers every aspect of life and has been defined by the United Nations as follows (based on the 1948 Universal Declaration of Human Rights):

> *Human rights are rights inherent to all human beings, regardless of race, sex, nationality, ethnicity, language, religion, or any other status. Human rights include the right to life and liberty, freedom from slavery and torture, freedom of opinion and expression, the right to work and education, and many more. Everyone is entitled to these rights, without discrimination.*
> UNITED NATIONS, HTTPS://WWW.UN.ORG/EN/GLOBAL-ISSUES/HUMAN-
> RIGHTS

These are obviously very broad principles, but they can be applied effectively to maternity services.

---

**PRACTICE POINTS AND COFFEE BREAK ACTIVITY**

**Practice points:**

Human rights in the maternity services
- *Respect* everyone receiving care and treat them as an individual with *dignity* and *respect*.
- Use best *evidence* to inform discussions and care plans.

- Make *decisions* with service users and families, not for them.
- *Empower* service users and pregnant people to have *control* over their own bodies and experiences—pregnancy and birth happen to them not to caregivers.
- Be aware of our own *beliefs* and *biases*—acknowledge these but leave them to one side when giving care.
- Be *honest*—about decisions, options, and mistakes.

**Activity**

Looking at the United Nations definition, note down any other areas of maternity care where human rights play a part. Are there any particular groups who you feel might be at greater risk of having their human rights not met?

Communication is an integral part of how we relate to other humans and safeguard or undermine their human rights. As we have seen in relation to risk in the previous section, the language that experts use can sometimes be alienating and frightening, even if it is not intended to be. It can also lead to some people or groups of people being excluded from care and decision-making, which adversely affects their human rights. The relative power of the maternity service and therefore those working in it is contrasted with the powerlessness of those using it. The language we use can sometimes seem old-fashioned or professional to us but to women it can seem intimidating and even threatening. This applies not just to the word 'risk' but also to other ways we talk about processes and care. Astrup (2018) wrote a useful article with ideas for replacing negative or judgemental clinical language with more neutral terms which acknowledged the rights of individuals (see the resource list as the end of this chapter for more details and for details of the #renamingrevolution glossary). Simple examples include using people's names instead of referring to them by their room number or condition: 'Jess' instead of 'Room 8' or 'the twin woman'.

## Case Study

Midwife, student midwife, woman and partner in the room. The student midwife is performing a booking interview with support from the midwife.

*Student midwife:* So you are a multip … did you have a normal birth last time?

*Woman:* I had to have a C-section …

*Midwife:* It says on your record that you had a section for failure to progress.

*Woman:* I was in labour all night.

*Midwife:* You only got to 2 cm so technically you weren't actually in labour.

*Woman:* No, I suppose not.

*Partner:* She was in a lot of pain.

*Student midwife:* And then you had a PPH on the ward?

*Woman:* I don't really remember but I did feel ill for a long time afterwards. Do I have to have another section?

*Midwife:* You could certainly try for a VBAC—but you'll have to talk to our VBAC midwife.

**ACTIVITY**

- If you were the woman and partner in this scenario, how might you feel?
- Compare this conversation to the ideas in Astrup's paper. How could you change the language used by the midwife and the student midwife? Jot down some examples.
- How might changing the language affect the human rights of the woman and her partner?
- If you were the student, is there anything you would do differently?

# Complexity

Pregnancy, labour and birth are at the same time very simple and incredibly complex. The human body is, mostly, designed to conceive, to grow the foetus and then to birth it and nurture it. However, as we have already seen in this chapter, there is so much more going on than just the physical. To explain the many different factors and links which go to make up the childbearing year, 'complexity' seems a useful word. It allows us to appreciate the concretions between mind and body, social, cultural spiritual and psychological wellbeing, and the process of pregnancy and birth. At its best the word 'complexity' reminds us that we can't know and anticipate everything. Every person and every situation are unique—no two labours and births are the same. One person with four children will tell different stories of each of them.

However, although an awareness of complexity is powerful and a useful corrective to taking things for granted, the maternity services have highjacked the word to use in quite specific circumstances. NICE used it in 2010 in their Guidelines discussing *Pregnancy and complex social factors: a model for service provision for pregnant women with complex social factors.* Their examples of complex social factors included pregnant teenagers, women who abused drugs or alcohol, and asylum seekers. At the time the Guidance was seen as useful recognition that women's experiences of pregnancy and birth were more than their physical situation. Complexity had previously been associated with multiple medical or obstetric issues rather than considering broader issues.

**QUICK REFLECTION**

Think about how the words 'complex' and 'complexity' are used in your area of practice.

- What sort of issues and circumstances do they cover?
- How do you think women and pregnant people feel about the description of 'complex' about them or their care?

When we communicate it is important to think about what we mean when we talk about complexity and the effect that this might have on the person hearing their situation or circumstance described as 'complex'. We may feel that it is a neutral phrase, but service users may find it threatening or a source of anxiety. We also need to be aware of the difference between 'complicated' and 'complex'. Murray Enkin (2006) wrote about the difference between 'simple', 'complicated' and 'complexity' in maternity care. He described learning to suture an episiotomy as 'simple'; you learn how to do it and the techniques hold true in any situation. Managing an obstetric emergency is 'complicated'; you need expertise, skill and flexibility but there is a clear link between any actions taken and the outcome. In contrast Enkin described 'complexity' as the simple things like delivering a baby—each time is different and unique and must be appreciated as such. This is not to say that things will go wrong but it reminds us that there are a lot of interlinked processes and circumstances which make up labour and birth. It is important to be aware that 'complexity' doesn't just become another word for 'pathology' or 'difficulty' and that it doesn't end up turning every element of pregnancy into a problem to be managed (Davies, 2012). At its best it should help to keep us humble in the face of things we cannot always predict or control, and give us the confidence to communicate to women and families how multifaceted pregnancy and birth really are.

## Uncertainty

One of the most challenging aspects of communication around pregnancy and birth is the uncertain nature of the experience and the way that we try to acknowledge or minimise that uncertainty. The old phrase 'birth is only normal in retrospect', which is often used to justify interventions is, at its heart, talking about the uncertainty of the process. One of the reasons that biomedical models of care have developed in maternity care is to try and reduce areas of uncertainty—and therefore of potential 'risk'. Midwives and other caregivers often struggle philosophically with uncertainty—with the unknowness of pregnancy and birth. We seek to organise, label and control it using technology such as ultrasound scanning, charts such as partograms and surveillance through vaginal examinations or foetal heart monitoring. We even seek to manage the uncertainty of women's coping skills by offering them analgesia and anaesthesia.

Our ability to cope with uncertainty is very individual—Page and Mander (2014) described how some midwives embraced the uncertainty of the process of labour, whereas as others felt destabilised by it and were constantly trying to anticipate issues or complications. In all cases midwives felt threatened by the idea of 'getting it wrong'—of making the wrong call in an uncertain situation where there were a variety of likely possibilities. This reminds us of Enkin's point in the previous section about the *complexity* of labour and birth.

Because we are so uncomfortable about uncertainty it makes it very difficult to communicate it. We want women and families to trust us and believe in us as professionals. This can make it very hard to admit that we don't know when asked a question or faced with a situation. We will often use strategies to avoid answering questions we can't answer such as answering a different question, which hasn't been asked, or minimising the situation. The clinical environment and the power imbalance between caregiver and care receiver can hamper honest dialogue. Let's look again at an aspect of the booking interview case study from earlier in the chapter:

### Case Study

*Student midwife*: And then you had a PPH on the ward?
*Woman*: I don't really remember but I did feel ill for a long time afterwards. Do I have to have another section?
*Midwife:* You could certainly try for a VBAC—but you'll have to talk to our VBAC midwife.

The woman wants to know if she will require another operative birth—the way she phrases it suggests that she is ambivalent or unhappy about the idea. The midwife does not directly answer 'yes' or 'no'—this would be difficult because at this point the midwife is uncertain about how labour and birth will proceed. The phrase 'certainly try' takes the doubt of the word 'try' (it might happen, it might not) and qualifies it with 'certainly' to make it seem definite. It doesn't exactly answer the woman's question—it answers a slightly different one in a way which seems clear and unambiguous but is quite vague. What else could the midwife have said? The midwife could have explored with the woman what prompted her question and therefore what answer she was looking for. They could have offered information about the chance of another section or other ways of birthing. The midwife could even have said 'I don't know' and explained why that was an appropriate answer.

Of course, it is not just caregivers who have to manage uncertainty—women and families are also dealing with the unknown and often in a much broader way. Health professionals have in mind the uncertainty around primarily the physical process. The pregnant person and family may be managing this but also wider social uncertainties around childcare, finances or employment or psychological ones around coping with pain, bonding or a changing sense of self. A study in the United States by Matthias (2009) found that midwives were generally better at supporting women through their uncertainties than doctors who were much more focused on biomedical issues. Midwives appeared better able to recognise and support women through what they were feeling. This suggests that if we are able to come alongside service users and work in partnership with them, then perhaps we need to be more honest in communicating our own uncertainty or the unknowness of pregnancy, labour and birth rather than attempting to give the impression that we know everything and can control everything.

## The Moral Dimension—Doing Good by Stealth?

So far, we have looked at concepts which have an explicit impact on how we practice and how we communicate our practice. However, there is another area of midwifery behaviour which is much more covert and which includes actions and omissions which are neither documented nor openly discussed. Over 20 years ago, midwife researcher Mavis Kirkham (1999) described the act of 'doing good by stealth'. This meant the actions of midwives in supporting other midwives to manage and survive in the care system without becoming disillusioned or burned out. More broadly it also meant midwives subverting technocratic norms of surveillance and intervention during labour and birth to give women a more physiological experience. Scamell and Stewart (2014) have explored this behaviour in relation to vaginal examinations performed by midwives. They identified that midwives might undertake examinations which they did not document (described as the 'quickie' or 'midwives VE') and which they did not necessarily gain explicit consent for. They also described midwives underestimating cervical dilation, particularly when women were on the borderline between the latent and active phases of labour or between first and second stage. Midwives explained their actions as supporting service users because whatever the risk-based rules said, they knew from experience that they did not need medical surveillance and intervention. Ethically they might argue that the end—the chance of a normal birth—justifies the means—covert interventions.

### QUICK REFLECTION

- Have you ever 'done good by stealth' in practice?
- Why did you do it?
- How did you communicate it to the care receiver and to other caregivers?
- How do you feel reflecting back—would you do the same again?

Scamell and Stewart noted that sometimes midwives explained their subterfuge to women but at other times they did not. It could be argued that this behaviour and the lack of open communication around it is a necessary response to a system that is very rigid and prioritises minimisation of risk over acceptance of uncertainty or complexity or even the human rights of pregnant people. However, it is not hard to see that undertaking actions which are not honestly agreed to or communicated carries its own risks and ethical uncertainties. It reminds us of the challenges of working and communicating in many maternity care systems.

## Conclusion

Specific chapters in the next sections of this book will explore aspects of communication in practice. This chapter has helped to set the scene by examining some of the broad issues and ideas that underpin how we care and communicate in the maternity services. We have considered what health communication is and what it means to juggle technical information, social support and care planning in a way that is kind and respectful. The chapter has explored some of the specific elements of health communication as they relate to the childbearing year—risk, human rights, complexity and uncertainty. It has examined what these ideas are and how they influence what and how we communicate with care receivers. It is impossible to say unambiguously 'this is how we should talk about risk', for example, because all these areas are slippery concepts which everyone sees and responds to differently. Instead this chapter has highlighted some of the issues in communicating these concepts together with suggestions about how we can increase our self-awareness when communicating them. It is also important to remember that these topics are not static—they constantly shift and so must our responses to them. New ideas and approaches may in the future supersede them and if this chapter tells us anything it is that we must remain open, honest, responsive and flexible in our communication with care receivers and other caregivers.

### References

Cheyne, H., Abhyankar, P., & Williams, B. (2012). Elective induction of labour: The problem of interpretation and communication of risks. *Midwifery*, 28, 412–415.

Coxon, K., Scamell, M., & Alaszewski, A. (2012). Risk, pregnancy and childbirth: What do we currently know and what do we need to know? An editorial. *Health, Risk and Society*, 14(6), 503–510.

Cross, R., Davis, S., & O'Neil, I. (2017). *Health communication theoretical and critical perspectives*. Polity Press.

Davies, L. (2012). Clinical complexity: The Emperor's new clothes? *Essentially MIDIRS*, 3(6), 17–22.

Enkin, M. (2006). Beyond evidence; the complexity of maternity care. *Birth*, 33(4), 265–269.

Kirkham, M. (1999). The culture of midwifery in the National Health Service in England. *Journal of Advanced Nursing*, 30(3), 732–739.

Lokugamage, A. U., & Pathberiya, S. D. C. (2017). Human rights in childbirth, narratives and restorative justice: A review. *Reproductive Health*, 14, 17.

Matthias, M. S. (2009). Problematic integration in pregnancy and childbirth: Contrasting approaches to uncertainty and desire in obstetric and midwifery care. *Health Communication, 24*(1), 60–70.

NHS England, (2016). *Better births. Improving outcomes of maternity services in England. A five year forward view for maternity care.* NHS England.

Page, M., & Mander, R. (2014). Intrapartum uncertainty: A feature of normal birth, as experienced by midwives in Scotland. *Midwifery, 30*, 28–35.

Sarangi, S., & Gilstad, H. (2014). Midwives communicative expertise in obstetric ultrasound encounters. Chapter 33. In H. E. Hamilton & W. S. Chou (Eds.), *The Routledge handbook of language and health communication.* Routledge.

Scamell, M., & Stewart, M. (2014). Time, risk and midwife practice: The vaginal examination. *Health, Risk & Society, 16*(1), 84–100.

Smith, V., Devane, D., & Murphy-Lawless, J. (2012). Risk in maternity care: A concept analysis. *International Journal of Childbirth, 2*(2), 126–135.

Waters, E. A., McQueen, A., & Cameron, L. D. (2014). Perceived risk and health risk communication. Chapter 3. In H. E. Hamilton & W. S. Chou (Eds.), *The Routledge handbook of language and health communication.* Routledge.

## Resources

Astrup, J. (2018). The language of labour. *Midwives Magazine.* https://www.rcm.org.uk/news-views/rcm-opinion/the-language-of-labour/

Mobbs, N., Williams, C., & Weeks, A.D. Humanising birth: Does the language we use matter? https://blogs.bmj.com/bmj/2018/02/08/humanising-birth-does-the-language-we-use-matter/

*These two papers both explore the use of language by health professionals: the first concentrates on midwives and the second on obstetric doctors. The papers explore the impact that insensitive language or jargon can have on service users and families. The papers also include suggestions of problematic language and how this can be adapted to become more person-centred, kind and respectful.*

Birthrights: https://www.birthrights.org.uk/

*Birthrights is a UK-based charity which was started in 2013 to promote human rights across the childbearing year. Their mission statement says that 'Birthrights is dedicated to ensuring women and birthing people receive the respect and dignity they deserve in pregnancy and childbirth.' Their website is a useful source of information on human rights issues around pregnancy and birth. They also conduct research and campaigns around specific issues—including, for example, dignity in childbirth, racial injustice and COVID-19.*

Peanut. The #RenamingRevolution https://www.peanut-app.io/blog/renaming-revolution-glossary

*This online resource has been developed by women in response to the judgemental and negative language often used in the medical and maternity services. It was developed after a service user in the United States posted a video on social media discussing how the use of the term 'geriatric mother' made her feel as a pregnant woman in her 30s.*

United Nations. (1948). *Universal declaration of Human Rights.* https://www.un.org/en/about-us/universal-declaration-of-human-rights

*This document, first published in 1948, sets out the core international beliefs and expectations about human rights in all areas of life. It is a useful foundation to thinking about human rights in childbearing and about the role and rights of caregivers. Ideas about dignity and respect from the Declaration underpin specific professional regulations—such as the UK Nursing and Midwifery Code. (2018). Professional standards of practice and behaviour for nurses, midwives and nursing associates. (https://www.nmc.org.uk/standards/code/).*

WRISK. https://wrisk.org/research-and-engagement/

*The WRISK project is a collaboration between the British Pregnancy Advisory Service (BPAS) and Heather Trickey at the School of Social Sciences at Cardiff University. Working with stakeholders from a wide range of disciplines, the project draws on women's experiences to understand and improve the development and communication of risk messages in pregnancy. The project is funded by the Wellcome Trust.*

# PART 2

# Responsive Communication

# CHAPTER 6

# Culturally Competent Communication

Fawzia Zaidi

## Introduction

Being able to communicate effectively with childbearing women and people is critical to understanding their bio-, psycho- and socio-cultural needs for them to receive the best possible person-centred care. Midwives are increasingly caring for people from diverse backgrounds; however, such diversity can make communication challenging since people from different backgrounds have different beliefs, behaviours, languages and meaning for words. The term 'culture' is often used synonymously with ethnicity and race. This chapter uses the term more broadly to encompass people who share common experiences that shape their understanding of the world. It can include groups that they are born in to, such as an ethnic group or socio-economic class, as well as groups that they have become a part of, such as transgender or disability groups. They may even move socio-economic class.

Intercultural communication is a process in which childbearing women, people and midwives from various cultural backgrounds interact with each other. Moreover, it is based on an understanding of their unique respective cultures (Yakar & Alpar, 2018). National policy (NHS England Patient and Public Participation and Insight Group, 2016), guidelines (Public Health England (PHE), 2017) and professional regulation (NMC, 2018) underscore effective person-centred communication. This approach encompasses the core values of respect, kindness, honesty and dignity as well as the principles of empowerment and treating people as individuals. These core values are reflected throughout the NMC Code (2018) and underpin effective communication. Yet evidence suggests that health care workers are ill-equipped to communicate efficiently across diverse cultural groups (Fair et al., 2020; Malouf et al., 2017; Zeeman et al., 2019). Poor intercultural communication within health care can lead to poor engagement with care plans, dissatisfaction with care, misunderstandings and poorer health outcomes.

**QUICK REFLECTION**

Think back to a time when you found yourself in a situation where you could not communicate with the majority group or population. How did that make you feel?

 

This chapter will consider the provision of respectful, person-centred communication with childbearing women, people and their families from diverse groups. It will include people with a neurodiversity, individuals with a sensory disability, and ethnic minority and lesbian, gay, bisexual, transgender, queer or questioning (LGBTQ+) groups. It will critically explore how personal and structural biases within maternity services are expressed during communication and can be mitigated by developing and applying the main attributes that underpin intercultural competent care. Accordingly, it will demonstrate how development of the attributes of cultural *awareness*, cultural *knowledge* and cultural *sensitivity* can support midwives in their intercultural communication. Consequently, it is anticipated that authentic respectful, trusting, person-centred relationships can be established resulting in better health outcomes and satisfaction for people and their families as well as increased job satisfaction for midwives.

# Cultural Awareness

**ATTRIBUTES OF CULTURAL AWARENESS**

Being aware of the presence of cultures different from one's own as well as the ability to recognise prejudice, discrimination, stereotypes and inequalities (Campinha-Bacote, 2002; Papadopoulos, 2006).

**Case Study**

Robbie is on a weekend break with her partner Grace when their membranes ruptured, and contractions started shortly after. They attend the labour ward, are unbooked in your unit and do not have their maternity records. You introduce yourself to Robbie and Grace and take them into a labour room. Along the way you ask Robbie how they are feeling. Grace is animated, loud and excited. She says it's been a nightmare trying to find the hospital and then having to find a parking space. Robbie climbs onto the bed, is quiet and anxious. As you move around the room you notice that Robbie's eyes follow you. As you attempt to take the history, Robbie looks towards Grace who then provides the answers. You sense that something is amiss.

**QUICK REFLECTION**

- How do you perceive disability?
- How do you perceive people seeking asylum?
- How do you perceive same-sex couples?
- How do you perceive people who are rude and brusque?
- What do these perceptions tell you about the lenses you use to view others?

It is anticipated that the elements of communication that recognise and take account of differences between midwives, women and people with respect to culture, values and beliefs can play a crucial role in reducing health inequities in the quality of midwifery care. Regrettably, health inequities amongst ethnic minority groups, LGBTQ+ groups and those with disabilities persist and can result from bias that is enacted at a personal and/or organisational level (Fernandez Turienzo et al., 2021; Rogers et al., 2017; Zeeman et al., 2019). The first step towards developing competent intercultural communication is for midwives to address their own biases as well as those within their organisation.

It is easier to converse with people who have similar social norms, beliefs and behaviours; however, when there are differences, communication can be awkward and difficult even if both parties speak English as their first language. Differences in ethnicity, gender self-identification, sexual orientation and disability identification may impact the values, beliefs and communication styles that each person brings to the interaction. This can result in misunderstandings and preclude the development of a trusting relationship. Intercultural communication therefore demands an intercultural awareness, acceptance and respect for differences between self and others. The reflection above reveals how we may see others through lenses coloured by our own cultural identity and beliefs. This ethnocentric bias, whether unconscious or conscious, can position the self as the archetype and judge others in comparison to this standard. It may be expressed as attitudes of superiority and/or hostility during intercultural interactions and can be a significant barrier to effective communication, giving rise to stereotypes, prejudice and discrimination.

As an adjunct to ethnocentrism, stereotypes are oversimplified perceptions or beliefs harboured about others which are founded on previously formed attitudes or opinions. These beliefs may or may not be true. They can be either positive or negative but are mostly negative. Negative stereotypes such as Black women and people have a low pain threshold in labour can direct midwives to communicate less effectively. The conversation can be less woman- and person-centred in that they may not be given the time or opportunity to discuss the nature of their pain. In addition, the midwife may not embark on a productive conversation about methods for pain relief. Similarly, body language such as not making eye contact with an

LGBTQ+ woman or person can also communicate a stereotype or a hostile message about that person. Often referred to as 'microaggressions', these examples of assertions and behaviour may leave the woman or person feeling frightened, isolated and undermined. Look at the case study and answer the following questions to see how stereotypes can operate:

- What assumptions did you make about Robbie and Grace in the scenario?
- What was informing your assumptions?
- How could your assumptions influence your interaction with Robbie and Grace?

Prejudice, like stereotypes, can also be positive or negative; however, it is generally referred to as a preconceived, usually unfavourable, evaluation or classification of another person based on a perceived personal characteristic of that person. A person who thinks that migrant Muslims or Eastern Europeans are terrorists or criminals, or that LGBTQ+ people should not be allowed to have children, is expressing a prejudice. Of course, there is no evidence that migrant Muslims or Eastern Europeans are more inclined to terrorist or criminal activities or of poor-quality parenting in LGBTQ+ couples; however, having a racist or homophobic mindset can lead to discriminatory behaviour. This is an intentional form of prejudice that hinders intercultural communication as it may involve unfavourable treatment or care and/or deny equal treatment or care to people. This could, for example, include not providing a professional interpreter for migrants with limited or no English or inappropriate questioning of LGBTQ+ people that is not related to care.

It can be difficult to accept that we may have prejudices especially because we have chosen to work in a caring profession; however, regardless of how we feel about ethnocentrism and prejudice, studies have shown that we are all susceptible to biases based on cultural stereotypes that are ingrained in our belief systems through socialisation from an early age (Bowler, 1993; Fitzgerald & Hurst, 2017). Developing self-awareness of our own cultural identity and beliefs along with a willingness to challenge and transform any biases is the first step towards building strong and trusting person-centred relationships with women and people. Becoming self-aware through critical reflection does not necessarily prevent biases; it does, however, make us more conscious of our personal biases.

## REDUCING BIAS

### Perspective Taking of the 'Other'

Returning to the scenario, imagine Robbie is a partially deaf trans man.
- How do you think he feels meeting you for the first time?
- What thoughts come to mind?
- What are you worried about?
- What are you excited about?

**Individuating—individual Identification of a Woman/Person Who Is Not 'Other'**
Are you focusing on Robbie's gender self-identification and disability identity?
Try and set aside or replace any assumptions so that you can get to know
Robbie as he is: an abstract artist who has exhibited widely. This is his first
pregnancy, and he is anxious because he is in an unfamiliar town and hospital
being cared for by someone that he has never met before.

**QUICK REFLECTION**

Can you identify any noninclusive language from the antenatal booking history
in your place of work?

Not all biases take place at a personal level. So-called egalitarian structures within maternity services such as policies, practices and systems also have the potential to discriminate against women and people. Such structures apply to everyone in the same way and are therefore considered fair. They can, however, disadvantage women and people with a protected characteristic such as race, gender reassignment, sexual orientation and disability, leading to indirect discrimination. Examples of how discrimination can play out during communication include the practice of identifying ethnicity at the antenatal booking visit. The Office for National Statistics (ONS), which has 18 groupings, is the tool that is generally used. While the data collected can help to assess risk, examine inequalities and access to services, the tool does have some drawbacks. For example, all African ethnic groups are combined despite Africa being a large and diverse continent with many different cultures. This underscores homogeneity when it does not exist. Furthermore, where an ethnic group is not represented, women and people are invited to choose 'other', which only reinforces difference. Another example is the bias towards heteronormativity in maternity settings. This is expressed through heterosexist language and options that are reflected in standardised forms such as the antenatal booking history and unconsciously communicated during the interaction. Organisational exclusions which assume that heterosexual families are the norm render LGBTQ+ partnerships and family constellations as socially invisible. Lastly, English-only signage in maternity units with a high immigrant population may be unconsciously sending the message that non-English-speaking women and people are not welcome.

Self-awareness is critical during the interaction. A self-aware midwife can discern how their personal biases may affect an interaction and attempt to manage them. Lastly, midwives need to be aware of how the language used in organisational structures can be biased against women and people from diverse groups. When personal and organisational biases are consciously or unconsciously communicated during interaction it can disempower women and people, removing their dignity and respect. The section on Cultural Sensitivity will explore how language can be modified to be inclusive.

**PRACTICE POINTS**

- Communication with women and people is influenced by individual culture.
- We are all susceptible to biases based on cultural stereotypes that are ingrained in our belief systems through socialisation from an early age.
- To mitigate stereotyping, midwives should develop self-awareness and challenge and transform any biases that may affect their communication with women and people from diverse groups.
- Reflect on and address organisational structures that perpetuate discrimination.

# Cultural Understanding

**ATTRIBUTES OF CULTURAL UNDERSTANDING**

Cultural understanding involves having information and an understanding of different cultures such as health beliefs and behaviours, as well as other components such as historical, political, social and economic factors (Papadopoulos, 2006; Suh, 2004).

The previous section proposed that midwives develop self-awareness to mitigate personal and organisational biases with the goal of building trusting relationships during interaction. This section will explore the concept of historical, socio-political and cultural understanding as one of the strategies for gaining trust and creating an instant rapport and connection to women and people from diverse groups. A lack of cultural understanding can cause fear and anxiety about communicating with women and people from diverse groups. Furthermore, it can also heighten negative attitudes towards them. The merits and limitations of possessing 'facts' about different cultural groups will also be examined alongside nonverbal communication behaviours that have potential for cross-cultural misunderstanding.

**QUICK REFLECTION**

- Do you know your local population?
- How many are from diverse groups?
- What are the social determinants of health in people from these diverse groups?
- What languages are spoken?

The definition implies that culture, historical, social, political and economic contexts are closely related. It suggests that midwives should possess knowledge and understanding of diverse cultures as well as the social context and circumstances in which women and people live, such as deprivation, exclusion, discrimination and stigma, and how these challenges might impact their communication. Lastly, women's and people's trust of and how they communicate with midwives may also be influenced by historical and political factors. Examples include the historical inhuman treatment of Black Americans such as the forced sterilisation of women based on their ethnicity up until the 1970s (Wheeler & Bryant, 2017). Until recently people with a disability were perceived as abnormal (Walsh-Gallagher et al., 2013) and people in same-sex relationships were considered to have a mental illness (Royal College of Psychiatrists, 2014). Stigma, discrimination and exclusion may have a significant impact on the lives of people across these groups. Despite a succession of legislation as well as national and local policies aimed at protecting individuals from these groups from discrimination, subtle discrimination persists. This can lead to a justified mistrust of people who have professional power and control (such as midwives) that can be reflected through their communication. Demonstrating understanding of historical and socio-political factors during communication conveys insight and empathy into the impact of the person's lived experiences. Moreover, it may counteract any exclusion, discrimination and stigma that they may have experienced in their previous health care encounters.

Certainly, the acquisition of cultural knowledge can reduce any anxieties about interacting with women and people from diverse backgrounds; however, cultures are not uniform. Significantly, a 'one type' of woman or person from a particular cultural group does not exist. There will be variations in attitudes, beliefs, behaviours and socio-economic status within and between cultural groups. Thus a focus on generalised beliefs and behaviours can result in stereotyping. This takes away the ability to understand the person as an individual, thereby undermining a person-centred relationship. It is suggested that any existing and future knowledge can be used as a point of reference to check understanding, but ultimately any cultural knowledge should be used with self-awareness, sensitivity and competence.

Instead of a focus on facts, Teal and Street (2009) propose that health care professionals are situationally aware. This involves being attentive to women and people by paying attention to the subtleties during communication, such as facial expressions and tone of voice. It is therefore proposed that self-awareness of cultural sensitivities coupled with an understanding of how nonverbal and paralanguage features are used and interpreted alongside good manners can be more effective during interactions. It can help to recognise and mitigate misunderstandings caused by incorrect assumptions and uneasiness due to cultural differences.

**QUICK REFLECTION**

- What are the characteristics of good manners?
- What factors impact good manners?
- What are the consequences of bad manners?

The way in which individuals use nonverbal signs such as personal space, touch, eye contact, facial expressions and gestures along with how they ascribe meaning to them in their everyday nonverbal communications is significantly influenced by culture. The amount of personal space that people are comfortable with varies from person to person and with the situation. Sitting close to a person may be regarded as an act of friendliness by some but threatening to others. The level of closeness during conversation may also be influenced by gender. Some ethnic minority women and people may feel more comfortable conversing in close proximity if the midwife is of the same gender. By contrast, some individuals with a neurodiversity may unintentionally invade the personal space of others. They may also be susceptible to sensory overload in their personal space (Pohl et al., 2020). Competing sensory input such as noise from visitors and crying babies, smells and lights may trigger a state of irritability, restlessness and anxiety leading to difficulty in focusing on what is being discussed. Personal space and touch are closely related. The nature of midwifery practice is highly sensory. Touch is frequently used by midwives to convey empathy and comfort, especially during labour; however, individuals in this group may not be comfortable with this practice. Preferences for physical space and touch should be ascertained and respected.

Body language such as eye contact, facial expressions and gestures are used to complement verbal communication. The way in which body language is used can denote interest and mirroring the person's facial expression can signal empathy. Using these features is invaluable, especially in situations where there is a language barrier or where the individual is deaf. There may, however, be situations where the midwife and person may misread each other's intentions. For example, some people with a neurodiversity may have difficulties in interpreting other people's facial expressions and gestures. They may also find eye contact uncomfortable and may lower their gaze or direct their attention away from the person who is speaking. In a similar way, direct eye contact is deemed disrespectful in some Asian cultures and some men may lower their gaze as a sign of respect if speaking to a female midwife. Lastly, midwives may not be able to read the facial expressions of Muslim people who are in full burqa. It is crucial that gestures are used with caution, facial expressions remain nonjudgemental, and eye contact should not be fixed or prolonged.

A paralanguage consists of variations in speech, such as voice quality, volume, tempo, pitch, nonfluencies (e.g., uh, um, ah), laughing, yawning, nodding and so on.

These nuances are used unconsciously to convey meaning. Nodding in particular shows interest and active listening. Paralanguage features cannot effectively cross cultural barriers, and a feature that means one thing in one culture can mean something else in another culture, giving rise to misunderstandings. For example, if a person speaks loudly, they may be perceived as being angry or aggressive; however, raising one's voice is common among many cultural groups to convey sincerity. Some ethnic minority groups and people with a neurodiversity may have difficulties in interpreting the nuances within conversations. Individuals from the latter group may also appear to be ill-mannered due to their constant interruptions and perceived interrogations; however, they may have problems processing verbal information due to sensory hypersensitivity leading to sensory overload (Pohl et al., 2020). Neurodiversity is an invisible disability and the behaviours of individuals with this condition may be incorrectly interpreted.

### QUICK REFLECTION

- Returning to the scenario, what knowledge do you think you need to communicate effectively with Robbie and Grace?
- What nonverbal behaviours might you need to consider when communicating with Robbie and Grace?

## Cultural Sensitivity

### ATTRIBUTES OF CULTURAL SENSITIVITY

Cultural sensitivity entails the development of interpersonal relationships with women and people and an equal partnership. It utilises one's knowledge and understanding and involves trust, empathy, acceptance, respect and adapting. If this is not achieved, health care professionals are in danger of using their power in an oppressive way (Chen & Young, 2012; Papadopoulos, 2006).

### PRACTICE POINTS

- A focus on surface-level cultural facts can result in stereotyping and cause offence.
- An understanding of historical and socio-political factors conveys insight and empathy into the impact of the person's lived experiences.
- Situational awareness of own and other's body language and paralanguage can mitigate misinterpretations and behaviours that may cause offence.

Cultural sensitivity employs the qualities of cultural awareness and understanding, as discussed in the previous sections. It is therefore a progressive process in which a person can effectively transform their cognitive and behavioural patterns shifting from ethnocentric stages to ethno-relative stages (Kalamatianou et al., 2020). The latter leads to an acceptance of and respect for cultural differences as evidenced by adapting one's behaviour and language so as not to cause offence during communication. Thus cultural sensitivity is an emotional feature of intercultural communication. If prejudice persists, there is a risk of midwives misusing their power to discriminate against women and people from diverse groups. This section will explore language and communication that is sensitive to the influences of the culture of people from diverse backgrounds.

> **QUICK REFLECTION**
>
> What sensitivities will you need to consider when communicating with Robbie and Grace?

Women and people may experience a range of emotions during their childbearing journey. Their feelings can range from excitement and happiness to fear, vulnerability and anxiety. Sensitive intercultural communication is therefore an essential component of midwifery care as they navigate this rollercoaster of emotions. It involves creating a welcoming environment by engaging in behaviours that demonstrate sensitivity and caring. This includes listening closely and showing interest, empathy and genuineness (Tucker et al., 2011) while being respectful and nonjudgemental. Such an approach is important in empowering women and people to make and confidently communicate their personal preferences. Conversely, insensitive communication can lead to anxiety, mistrust and disengagement with maternity services.

Language can dehumanise. When meeting women and people for the first time, it is crucial to respect and be sensitive to the language that people use to describe themselves, their parenting role and their family structure and to reflect it back during communication. This reinforces and makes visible their identity and parenting role. It also prevents harm to relationships before they even start. The Cultural Awareness section highlighted how LGBTQ+ individuals may experience indirect discrimination because of heteronormative maternity services and negative attitudes and behaviour from health care professionals. Heteronormative ideology assumes that 'parents' are composed of a man and a woman. This assumption about family structure can result in the insensitive use of heterosexist language when communicating with individuals who self-identify as LGBTQ+. It further undermines their identities as parents. An example of this is asking about the father or referring to the nonbiological mother or co-parent in a lesbian partnership as the sister or friend.

Sex-based language such as 'woman' and 'mother' and feminine pronouns (she/her) are widely used in midwifery. More recently, there has been a shift towards the use of gender-neutral or nonsexed language during pregnancy, birth and lactation. The principal aim underlying this shift is sensitivity to and acknowledgement of individuals who are biologically female (sex) but do not identify as women due to their gender identity (inner sense of self) (Gribble et al., 2022). The debate on replacing sex-based language with gender-neutral language and/or using gender-additive language (e.g., women and people) to reflect inclusivity is contentious and is subject to an ongoing discourse. The reader is directed to the work of Gribble et al. (2022), who present a comprehensive discussion of the unintended consequences of such replacements en masse. This is especially in relation to vulnerable groups (such as those with limited English) where obfuscation of communication can lead to misunderstandings. The author of this chapter does not advocate avoiding gender in one-to-one communication altogether, rather any replacements should reflect the gender identity and family structure of the individual and the context. For example, with respect to family structure, saying 'parents' instead of 'mums' and 'dads' when facilitating antenatal classes helps to include more family structures.

Inclusive language is not fixed and keeping pace can be bewildering. There may be concerns about what words to use or of using outdated words to describe individuals and groups of people. Although Box 6.1 presents some helpful pointers for using inclusive language, the reader is also prompted to find out about inclusive language that is used within their communities and their place of work.

**QUICK REFLECTION**

How would you describe a woman who says that she was born in England, but her parents are from Guyana? Her mother is Chinese, and her father is South Asian.

It is natural to be curious about the lives of people from diverse groups; however, this can result in the inappropriate questioning of people from these groups. Personal questions should be asked in a sensitive manner and only if it is relevant for their care. Furthermore, the reasons for asking such questions should be explained. For example, asking about ethnicity at the antenatal booking to assess for potential genetic risk factors such as haemoglobinopathies may be perceived as racist or as a way of checking the person's immigration status. Asking trans men about hormone therapy is important with respect to stopping testosterone during pregnancy and when to reinitiate it. Similarly, asking them about surgery is significant when considering mode of delivery and its impact on gender dysmorphia. Unfortunately, they may have been asked these personal and intrusive questions out of context in the past. This may have made them feel that they were an object of curiosity. Innocuous inquisitiveness about the experiences of people from diverse groups can be researched outside of the clinical interaction.

## BOX 6.1 ■ Helpful Pointers for Using Inclusive Language

### Gender
- If there is any doubt regarding how an individual self-identifies the best course of action is to inquire.
- Call individuals by the name that they use and not their legal name. Using the latter implies that you do not recognise their preferred name as 'real'.
- Use self-identified gender pronouns.
- Avoid using nongendered language to describe someone who has said that they use gendered language as this disrespects their choice of language.
- If they have fought to have their gender identity acknowledged, being referred to solely by nongendered language when they have indicated otherwise can cause harm and gender dysphoria.
- Misgendering can cause distress and reduce trust. To avoid further embarrassment to both parties, it is advisable to promptly apologise, correct the mistake and move on.
- The childbearing parent and their partner will identify how they wish to be addressed (e.g., pregnant person, birthing person, father, parent, co-parent).
- Find out and use the words that the individual uses to describe their body parts (e.g., chest instead of breast and genital opening instead of vagina), how it works (e.g., chest feeding instead of breastfeeding) and what it produces (e.g., human/chest milk instead of breastmilk).

(Brighton and Sussex University Hospitals NHS Trust, 2020; British Medical Association (BMA), 2016)

### Sexual Orientation
- Ask about and use their parenting names (e.g., mother, second mother, co-parent).

### Disability
- Allow individuals to define themselves (e.g., blind person, deaf person, neuro-divergent person). Put the person first. Use adjectives rather than nouns (e.g., person with a visual impairment, person with a hearing impairment, person with a neurodiversity).
- Listen to how the individual describes their impairment.

(BMA, 2016)

### Ethnicity
- Allow individuals to define themselves.
- The acronym BAME (Black, Asian and Minority Ethnic) is controversial as it indiscriminately amalgamates people from different geographical, social and cultural backgrounds. Furthermore, the first two letters emphasise skin colour (Khunti et al., 2020).
- Avoid using the term 'race'. When loaded with meaning, this word can define minority individuals as a negative. It suggests that there are inborn biological differences between ethnic groups (inferior/superior race).
- 'Person of colour' can be considered offensive because it combines all 'non-White' individuals together thereby undermining individual identity.
- 'Coloured' person is offensive. The word has long been connected with segregation, particularly in the United States, where Black people were separated from White people. This constituted racist behaviour.

Although midwives should consciously try to communicate with everyone with dignity and respect, the reality is that communication can be directed by perceptions and beliefs about who the person is and how they should be spoken to. This is one of the unintended consequences of stereotyping as discussed in the Cultural Awareness section. It can result in insensitive communication leading to misunderstandings and mistrust. For example, when communicating with people who speak limited or no English, or people with a sensory disability or neurodiversity, there can be a tendency to only talk to the accompanying person or to adjust one's style of speech. Unfortunately, the latter often includes talking loudly, altering the tone of one's voice or speaking really slowly. Talking in this way can come over as patronising or imply that the person has a learning disability.

When talking to people from the foregoing groups, it is important to offer them the same good manners and respect that are shown to others while attending to any cultural sensitivities. Such considerations may include:

- Finding out about a person's preferred method of communication and offering appropriate assistance. For example, people with a hearing impairment may prefer to use text or to lip read over signing. Interpreting services can also be offered, including to those with limited or no English language proficiency. These services will be discussed in the next section.
- Talking in an age-appropriate tone (not like talking to a child).
- Being patient and encouraging. Letting the person set the pace of the conversation so that they can process the verbal information. This is important with those who have a neurodiversity and those who are speaking English as their second language.
- Speaking clearly and directly to the person even if there is an interpreter present.
- Using short sentences to avoid ambiguity. People with a neurodiversity, for example, want clear information and no 'fluffy' language (Hampton et al., 2022).
- Avoiding questions that require a 'yes' or 'no' answer. In some ethnic minority cultures, it is awkward to answer negatively, so even if the correct answer is 'no', it will always be 'yes'; furthermore, they may answer 'yes' because they do not understand what is being asked and want to end the conversation (Schott & Henley, 1996). Asking an open-ended question that requires information is therefore more effective.
- Being mindful of witticisms. English humour may not be understood by migrant populations. In addition, people with a neurodiversity are often literal thinkers and may attach a different meaning to a joke, which can cause confusion.
- Avoiding euphemisms such as 'down there', 'waterworks' and 'the other end' (Bowler, 1993). These expressions are often substituted when referring to

anatomy that is considered embarrassing; however, people with limited English language proficiency may understand the individual words but not the context and hence the meaning.

- Avoiding closed questions to check understanding especially with those who have a hearing impairment or those with a neurodiversity or limited English. Repeating or summarising what the person has said confirms that what they have said has been understood. By contrast, asking them questions can check out their understanding.
- Using illustrations with caution as they may cause offence.

Specific sensitivities when communicating with people who have a sensory impairment include providing simple explanations that are not necessary with people who are not sensory impaired. For example, people with a vision impairment want to be told what is happening in the room, who is entering and leaving, and what is happening to them in that moment (Schildberger et al., 2017). It should not be assumed that people with a hearing impairment can lip read and even if they can, their ability to do so may be compromised when in pain or sleepy from analgesia (Schildberger et al., 2017). They are also less likely to have a working understanding of terms linked to childbirth (Luton et al., 2022).

**PRACTICE POINTS**

- Cultural insensitivity can lead to an unjust use of power.
- Avoid assumptions. Respect and use the language that women and people use to describe themselves, their parenting role and their family structure.
- Language and communication behaviours should be sensitive to the influences of the culture of women and people.

# Cultural Competence

**ATTRIBUTES OF CULTURAL COMPETENCE**

Cultural competency necessitates the integration of previously acquired awareness, knowledge and sensitivity and their use in the assessment of needs, clinical diagnosis and other caring skills. The ability to recognise and confront racism and other types of discrimination and oppressive conduct is a critical component of this stage (Papadopoulos, 2006).

The first part of the definition implies that culturally competent communication is not a separate attribute. It entails communicating with an awareness of personal and organisational biases, an understanding that historical and socio-cultural and political factors have important effects on behaviours, and having the ability to adapt one's own behaviour and communication to avoid causing offence. Ultimately, culturally competent communication can only be achieved if there is a genuine willingness to develop each of these attributes. Indeed, the previous section underscored the developmental qualities of cultural sensitivity as shifting from ethnocentric stages to ethnorelative stages (Kalamatianou et al., 2020). Reflection on and in action (Schon, 1987) is a powerful tool for developing culturally competent communication. The reflection in action can empower midwives to challenge and transform any biases and make changes to their communication style in future experiences. By contrast, the reflection on action requires a situational awareness (as discussed in the Cultural Understanding section), whereby subtleties during communication are recognised from previous experiences in action which may necessitate the need for adaptations; thus situational awareness is combined with action.

**QUICK REFLECTION**

Who would you contact if you need to access communication support for the following:
- A person with limited English language proficiency.
- A person who is deaf.

National policy (NHS England Patient and Public Participation and Insight Group, 2016) mandates access to 'accessible, inclusive information and communication support to all' (p. 5) in England. This includes information in alternative languages and formats such as audio, Braille, British Sign Language (BSL), easy read or large print as well as access to a professional interpreter. Teal and Street (2009), however, draw attention to how culturally competent communication can be delivered through an interpreter. Indeed, the author was unable to find studies which specifically evaluate the role of interpreters through the elements of cultural competence in a maternity or any health care setting. Nevertheless, professional interpreters are considered the gold standard and a range of interpretation services are offered. These include access to face-to-face professional interpreters, bilingual health care professionals and telephone translation services such as language line for those with limited or no English. It is proposed that an understanding of some of the issues associated with the different types of interpreters alongside some solutions (Box 6.2) will enable midwives to work alongside interpreters to deliver culturally competent communication.

**QUICK REFLECTION**

Returning to Robbie and Grace, what might you need to consider if using an interpreter?

When considering the use of an interpreter, it is critical to include women and people in the decision-making process regarding the type of interpreter (professional

## BOX 6.2 ■ Communication Support: Issues and Solutions

| Type of Communication Support | Issue | Solution |
| --- | --- | --- |
| Professional interpreters | Not knowing how to book an interpreter.<br>Choice of interpreter when discussing intimate or difficult matters.<br>Not knowing how to work with interpreters.<br>Confidentiality, especially if they are from the same community as the woman or person. | Find out how to book interpreters in your area of practice.<br>Consider the woman's/person's preferences with regards to the age, gender, religion, ethnic origin and characteristics of the interpreter.<br>Awareness training in BSL.<br>Training on the midwife–interpreter relationship. Treat the interpreter as a colleague and support them. Make clear the aim of the interpretation.<br>The professional interpreter needs to reassure the woman/person that they have training and experience and will uphold the principles of neutrality and integrity. |
| Bilingual health care professional | Limited language skills.<br>Lack of training in interpreting.<br>Limited knowledge of childbirth or terminology if not working in a maternity setting. | Try to avoid and only use in an emergency. |
| Telephone translation services | Not fully interactive.<br>Loss of nonverbal communication. | Use remote face-to-face interpreting. |

| Type of Communication Support | Issue | Solution |
|---|---|---|
| Family members | Distorted or biased translation. | Using a professional interpreter (with consent) gives some surety around quality, accuracy and confidentiality. |
| | Embarrassment in that the woman or person may be ashamed to discuss intimate issues, especially if the interpreter is a child. | |
| | The family member may not have a good understanding of English to communicate complex information. | It is advised that women and people be seen on their own at least once during their pregnancy to enable them to discuss sensitive issues that they may not be able to discuss in front of family members. |
| | Less likely to disclose sensitive issues such as alcohol and drug consumption, domestic abuse, mental health issues and sexually transmitted disease. | |
| Google Translate | Not recommended in maternity. | Use with caution. It has been found to be an initial communication tool in health care. |
| | Not trusted for important medical communication. | |

*BSL*, British Sign Language.
From Fair, F., Raben, L., Watson, H., Vivilaki, V., van den Muijsenbergh, M., Soltani, H., et al. (2020). Migrant women's experiences of pregnancy, childbirth and maternity care in European countries: A systematic review. *PLoS One, 15*, e0228378; Luton, M., Allan, H. T., & Kaur, H. (2022). Deaf women's experiences of maternity and primary care: An integrative review. *Midwifery, 104*, 103190; Rayment-Jones, H., Harris, J., Harden, A., et al. (2021). Project20: Interpreter services for pregnant women with social risk factors in England: What works, for whom, in what circumstances, and how? *International Journal for Equity in Health, 20*, 233.

interpreter, bilingual health care worker, family member) and mode of interpreting (face to face or telephone) in order to select the most appropriate interpreter. Many women and people may trust and feel secure using family members as interpreters. For example, women and people who are deaf felt that that they had been dependent on their relatives to speak for them as they grew up, and that they now lacked the confidence to speak for themselves (Luton et al., 2021).

Language-appropriate written information should not be used as a substitute for face-to-face communication. It can be given to reinforce the verbal information; however, it should be distributed with caution as access will be dependent on levels of literacy. For example, some women and people with limited English language proficiency may be nonreaders of their own language. Similarly, women and people who are deaf may have been educationally disadvantaged, resulting in lower levels of reading and writing skills than their hearing counterparts (Luton et al., 2022). Thus the language in any written material may need to be simplified so that it can be understood. Equally, a woman or person who is blind may not be able to read Braille. Any additional information can be given in an alternative format such as audio or via email. If using the latter, it is important to check that the person has the assisted technology or software which converts text to speech. Lastly, some women and people with a neurodiversity may find bright colours in leaflets difficult, leading to anxiety.

Culturally competent communication involves challenging discrimination as it happens. This can be at an informal level by interrupting an interaction between a colleague and a woman or person to prevent further harm or letting them know afterwards that their language or communication behaviour is unacceptable. Of course, this can be awkward and frightening and it may carry risks, especially if the colleague is in a senior position. If the behaviour persists, a formal route may have to be taken. Finally, midwives have the power to address noninclusivity by influencing and advocating for policies and guidelines that can have a positive impact on women and people from diverse groups.

**PRACTICE POINTS**

- Include the woman or person in the decision-making process with regards to type of interpreter and mode of interpreting.
- Work with and support interpreters to deliver culturally competent communication.
- Use written information with caution.
- Call out discrimination when you see it and challenge noninclusive policies and guidelines.

# Conclusion

This chapter has discussed respectful person-centred intercultural communication with women and people from diverse groups through the lens of cultural competence. It emphasises the development and application of the attributes of cultural awareness, understanding and sensitivity. This includes attending to personal and organisational biases, demonstrating an understanding of how historical and socio-political factors can impact the person's lived experiences, being mindful of language and communication behaviours that can cause offence, and calling out discriminatory language and behaviour. Culturally competent communication can only be achieved through continuous critical reflection alongside a genuine desire to develop each of the attributes.

---

**QUICK REFLECTION**

Having read this chapter and after communicating with a woman or person from a diverse group, reflect on the following:
- What were the barriers to communication?
- What knowledge did you draw on to facilitate communication?
- What adaptations did you have to make to ensure that communication was sensitive to the culture of the woman or person?
- What else facilitated you in your communication?
- What would you do differently in a similar situation?

---

## References

Bowler, I. (1993). 'They're not the same as us': Midwives' stereotypes of South Asian descent maternity patients. *Sociology of Health and Illness, 15,* 157–178.

Brighton and Sussex University Hospitals NHS Trust, (2020). *Gender inclusive language in perinatal services: Mission statement and rationale.* NHS.

British Medical Association, (2016). *A guide to effective communication: Inclusive language in the workplace.* British Medical Association. https://archive.org/details/2016BritishMedic alAssociationBMAGuideToEffectiveCommunication2016/page/n1/mode/2up. Accessed 21 December 2021.

Campinha-Bacote, J. (2002). The process of cultural competence in the delivery of healthcare services: A model of care. *Journal of Transcultural Nursing, 13*(3), 181–184.

Chen, G. M., & Young, P. (2012). Intercultural communication competence. In A. Goodboy & K. Shultz (Eds.), *Introduction to communication: Translating scholarship into meaningful practice* (pp. 175–188). Kendall-Hunt.

Fair, F., Raben, L., Watson, H., Vivilaki, V., van den Muijsenbergh, M., Soltani, H., & ORAMMA Team (2020). Migrant women's experiences of pregnancy, childbirth and maternity care in European countries: A systematic review. *PLoS One, 15*(2), e0228378. https://doi.org/10.1371/journal.pone.0228378.

Fernandez Turienzo, C., Newburn, M., Agyepong, A., Buabeng, R., Dignam, A., Abe, C., Bedward, L., Rayment-Jones, H., Silverio, S. A., Easter, A., Carson, L. E., Howard, L. M., & Sandall, J., & NIHR ARC South London Maternity and Perinatal Mental Health Research and Advisory Teams (2021). Addressing inequities in maternal health among women living in communities of social disadvantage and ethnic diversity. *BMC Public Health, 21,* 176. https://doi.org/10.1186/s12889-021-10182-4.

FitzGerald, C., & Hurst, S. (2017). Implicit bias in healthcare professionals: A systematic review. *BMC Medical Ethics, 18*(1), 19. https://doi.org/10.1186/s12910-017-0179-8.

Gribble, K. D., Bewley, S., Bartick, M. C., Mathisen, R., Walker, S., Gamble, J., Bergman, N. J., Gupta, A., Hocking, J. J., & Dahlen, H. G. (2022). Effective communication about pregnancy, birth, lactation, breastfeeding and newborn care: The importance of sexed language. *Frontiers in Global Women's Health, 3,* 818856.

https://www.frontiersin.org/article/10.3389/fgwh.2022.818856.doi:10.3389/
fgwh.2022.818856, ISSN2673-5059.

Hampton, S., Man, J., Allison, C., Aydin, E., Baron-Cohen, S., & Holt, R. (2022). A qualitative exploration of autistic mothers' experiences II: Childbirth and postnatal experiences. *Autism, 26*(5), 1165–1175. https://doi.org/10.1177/13623613211043701.

Kalamatianou, A., Spinthourakis, J. A., & Panagopoulos, E. (2020). The effectiveness of translanguaging language practices in bilingual education: A literature review. In B. Krzywosz-Rynkiewicz & V. Zorbas (Eds.), *Citizenship at a crossroads: Rights, identity, and education* (pp. 322–332). Charles University and Children's Identity and Citizenship European Association.

Khunti, K., Routen, A., & Pareek, M. (2020). The language of ethnicity. *BMJ, 371,* m4493. https://doi.org/10.1136/bmj.m4493.

Luton, M., Allan, H. T., & Kaur, H. (2022). Deaf women's experiences of maternity and primary care: An integrative review. *Midwifery, 104,* 103190. https://doi.org/10.1016/j.midw.2021.103190.

Malouf, R., Henderson, J., & Redshaw, M. (2017). Access and quality of maternity care for disabled women during pregnancy, birth and the postnatal period in England: Data from a national survey. *BMJ Open, 7*(7), p.e016757.

NHS England Patient and Public Participation and Insight Group (2016). *NHS England accessible information and communication policy.* nhse-access-info-comms-policy.pdf (england.nhs.uk). Accessed 20 October 2021.

NMC, (2018). *The code: Professional standards of practice and behaviour for nurses, midwives and nursing associates.* The Nursing and Midwifery Council. https://www.nmc.org.uk/standards/code/. Accessed 20 October 2021.

Papadopoulos, I. (2006). The Papadopoulos, Tilki and Taylor model for the development of cultural competency in nursing. In I. Papadopoulos (Ed.), *Transcultural health & social care: Development of culturally competent practitioners* (pp. 7–24). Churchill Livingstone.

Pohl, A. L., Crockford, S. K., Blakemore, M., Allison, C., & Baron-Cohen, S. (2020). A comparative study of autistic and non-autistic women's experience of motherhood. *Molecular Autism, 11*(1), 3. https://doi.org/10.1186/s13229-019-0304-2.

Public Health England. (2017). *Language interpretation: Migrant health guide.* Up-dated 2021. https://www.gov.uk/guidance/language-interpretation-migrant-health-guide. Accessed 30 August 2021.

Rayment-Jones, H., Harris, J., Harden, A., Silverio, S. A., Turienzo, C. F., & Sandall, J. (2021). Project20: Interpreter services for pregnant women with social risk factors in England: What works, for whom, in what circumstances, and how? *International Journal for Equity in Health, 20,* 233. https://doi.org/10.1186/s12939-021-01570-8.

Rogers, C., Lepherd, L., Ganguly, R., & Jacob-Rogers, S. (2017). Perinatal issues for women with high functioning autism spectrum disorder. *Women and Birth, 30*(2), e89–e95.

Royal College of Psychiatrists. (2014). *Royal College of Psychiatrists statement on sexual orientation. Position statement PS02/2014.* https://www.rcpsych.ac.uk/pdf/PS02_2014.pdf. Accessed 22 December 2021.

Schildberger, B., Zenzmaier, C., & König-Bachmann, M. (2017). Experiences of Austrian mothers with mobility or sensory impairments during pregnancy, childbirth and the puerperium: A qualitative study. *BMC Pregnancy and Childbirth, 17,* 201. https://doi.org/10.1186/s12884-017-1388-3.

Schon, D. (1987). *Educating the reflective practitioner: Towards a new design for teaching and learning in the professions.* Jossey Bass.

Suh, E. E. (2004). The model of cultural competence through an evolutionary concept analysis. *Journal of Transcultural Nursing, 15*(2), 93–102.

Teal, C. R., & Street, R. L. (2009). Critical elements of culturally competent communication in the medical encounter: A review and model. *Social Science and Medicine, 68*(3), 533–543. https://doi.org/10.1016/j.socscimed.2008.10.015.

Tucker, C. M., Marsiske, M., Rice, K. G., Nielson, J. J., & Herman, K. (2011). Patient-centered culturally sensitive health care: Model testing and refinement. *Health Psychology: Official Journal of the Division of Health Psychology, American Psychological Association, 30*(3), 342–350. https://doi.org/10.1037/a0022967.

Walsh-Gallagher, D., Mc Conkey, R., Sinclair, M., & Clarke, R. (2013). Normalising birth for women with a disability: The challenges facing practitioners. *Midwifery, 29*, 294–299. https://doi.org/10.1016/j.midw.2011.10.007.

Wheeler, S. M., & Bryant, A. S. (2017). Racial and ethnic disparities in health and health care. *Obstetrics and Gynecology Clinics of North America, 44*(1), 1–11. https://doi.org/10.1016/j.ogc.2016.10.001. PMID: 28160887.

Yakar, H. K., & Alpar, S. E. (2018). Intercultural communication competence of nurses providing care for patients from different cultures. *International Journal of Caring Sciences, 11*(3), 1396–1409.

Zeeman, L., Sherriff, N., Browne, K., McGlynn, N., Mirandola, M., Gios, L., Davis, R., Sanchez-Lambert, J., Aujean, S., Pinto, N., Farinella, F., Donisi, V., Niedźwiedzka-Stadnik, M., Rosińska, M., Pierson, A., Amaddeo, F., & Health4LGBTI Network. (2019). A review of lesbian, gay, bisexual, trans and intersex (LGBTI) health and healthcare inequalities. *European Journal of Public Health, 29*(5), 74–980. https://doi.org/10.1093/eurpub/cky226.

## Further Reading

Grant, L. (2015). *From here to maternity. Pregnancy and motherhood on the autism spectrum.* Jessica Kingsley Publishers.
> *Already the mother of five children, Lana Grant's late diagnosis of autism at the age of 38 transformed her experience in her sixth pregnancy. Based on her own experiences of the challenges and joys of pregnancy and motherhood, it gives insight into the unique challenges faced by mothers on the spectrum.*

Gribble, K. D., Bewley, S., Bartick, M. C., Mathisen, R., Walker, S., Gamble, J., Bergman, N. J., Gupta, A., Hocking, J. J., & Dahlen, H. G. (2022). Effective communication about pregnancy, birth, lactation, breastfeeding and newborn care: The importance of sexed language. *Frontiers in Global Women's Health, 3*, 818856. https://doi:10.3389/fgwh.2022.818856. https://www.frontiersin.org/article/10.3389/fgwh.2022.818856. ISSN2673-5059.
> *Highly recommended. This article contributes to the discourse on using replacement language and addresses the unintended consequences of replacing sexed language.*

Schott, J., & Henley, A. (1996). *Culture, religion and childbearing in a multiracial society. A handbook for health professionals.* Butterworth-Heinemann.
> *An excellent resource for understanding how culture and religion impact pregnancy and childbirth.*

World Health Organization. (2020) *Migration and health: Enhancing intercultural competence and diversity sensitivity.* https://www.who.int/europe/publications/i/item/9789289056632
> *This toolkit focuses on intercultural competence and diversity sensitivity in relation to refugees and migrants.*

## Websites

About Stonewall and our Diversity Champions programme. https://www.stonewall.org.uk/about-us/news/about-stonewall-and-our-diversity-champions-programme
> *Stonewall is a lesbian, gay, bisexual and transgender rights charity in the United Kingdom. It is the largest LGBT rights organisation in Europe.*

List of LGBTQ+ terms. https://www.stonewall.org.uk/help-advice/information-and-resources/faqs-and-glossary/list-lgbtq-terms#g
   *Glossary of LGBTQ+ terms from Stonewall.*

What is autism. https://www.autism.org.uk/advice-and-guidance/topics/what-is-autism
   *This is the website of the National Autistic Society.*

Deafblind UK | Supporting Deafblindness in the UK. https://deafblind.org.uk
   *Deafblind UK is a national charity that supports deafblind people and those with progressive sight and hearing loss. There is a range of communication resources for professionals.*

## *YouTube Videos*

Perspective taking. https://youtu.be/tqz7UcCgbLA
   *This video explains perspective taking.*

Stereotypes vs. prejudice vs. discrimination. https://youtu.be/6Hr2XpBc_B4
   *This video differentiates between stereotypes, prejudice and discrimination. It discusses important social psychological concepts and hypotheses related to each, including what causes them to arise in the first place.*

# CHAPTER 7

# Public Health

Jane Rooney

## Introduction

This chapter focuses on communication for one of the key roles of midwifery practice—supporting and delivering care around public health. Public health has been defined as 'the art and science of preventing disease, prolonging life and promoting health through the organised efforts of society' (Acheson, 1988). In simple terms, public health is an umbrella term which covers many different aspects of life-course health, with a core part focusing on personal, community and population contribution and action to improving health outcomes for all (Acheson, 1988).

Midwives are uniquely placed to deliver public health because of their one-to-one role in supporting people and families during the childbearing year. Effective public health can contribute to safe, high-quality outcomes for families (Department of Health, 2013a; Marshall et al., 2019). There is a greater emphasis now on embedding public health values as an integral part of the midwife's role, and this can be seen by the development of the recent NMC Standards for Proficiency (Meegan, 2020). Undergraduate curricula have now been changed to reflect the new standards, and midwives currently in practice will need to ensure that they update themselves accordingly. The widening of the midwife's role in public health is a recognition of the crucial part that they play in improving broader health outcomes for families.

---

**QUICK REFLECTION**

- What aspects of public health do I currently deliver on a daily or regular basis in my midwifery role?
- Where are my knowledge, skills and confidence at now in relation to these public health aspects?
- How does communication in these public health aspects shape the service that I deliver?

---

Throughout the childbearing continuum, at all stages and at all points along the maternity care timeline, midwives communicate with women, birthing people and families about a broad range of public health issues. This chapter considers the background to public health in midwifery and the key principles of communication. It will then use the example of smoking cessation to work through the range of communication techniques and tools which midwives can use to deliver and develop their practice. Although smoking is the example topic, the ideas and techniques are applicable and useful in all midwifery public health encounters.

## Challenges in Public Health Communication

Recent evidence suggests that midwives sometimes lack one or more of the essential communication elements (see Fig. 7.1) which are fundamental to delivering excellence in public health midwifery care (Gomez & Chilvers, 2017, p. 16). These can be overarching and related to our knowledge and skills in public health, or they can be specifically linked to working with a particular family or issue.

Some public health topics can be seen as more sensitive or difficult to communicate about, for example, obesity and diet, smoking cessation and mental health. A lack of midwifery confidence in tackling these public health issues may mean that opportunities to improve health are reduced or missed altogether.

It is often when we face difficulties in professional development that we feel less confident to address public health issues. This model helps us to continue to reflect on building these elements into our midwifery practice and will be used throughout the chapter to support development around public health communication.

As we can see from Fig. 7.1 there are personal and structural reasons why public health communication can be a challenge. In the context of a very busy service, a lack of time can have a significant impact on the quality of communication around

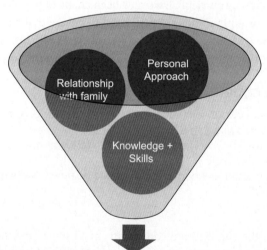

**Fig. 7.1**   The confidence model: essential communication elements for creating and utilising public health opportunities in midwifery care.

public health. It takes time and space to have sensitive, individualised conversations on challenging and personal topics. A lack of time can mean that conversations are rushed or skipped altogether. Fig. 7.2 illustrates some of the main structural challenges in supporting meaningful public health conversations.

Evidence does confirm that information, advice and support on public health issues can be actioned in a short time frame, but this can be difficult to balance alongside other elements of the midwife's role (Marshall et al., 2019). This 'brief intervention' approach has value, but for a number of sensitive issues such as obesity, midwives often feel as if more time is needed for them to feel confident in the conversation and any referrals and follow-up which may be offered (Crabbe & Hemingway, 2014; Gomez & Chilvers, 2017; Lawrence et al., 2020).

**COFFEE BREAK ACTIVITY**

Drawing on a recent practice experience, reflect on the three elements of the confidence model (Fig. 7.1).
- Which of these do you use the most?
- Which area do you find most challenging?
- What barriers may prevent the elements from functioning?
- What can you do to work on your confidence in using the different elements?

For the National Health Service (NHS) there is a focus on annual mandatory training, which includes several core elements deemed to be needed for safety and quality purposes. As public health in maternity covers such a wide remit, there is not the resource to cover all issues, and many are restricted to core elements such as infant feeding. Anything additional may be on a less frequent basis, or available as a nonmandatory refresher to maternity staff. Many students and qualified

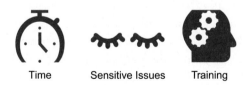

Time          Sensitive Issues          Training

Environment

**Fig. 7.2** Structural challenges to meaningful public health conversations.

midwives lack confidence (see Fig. 7.1) around public health communication due to this gap in education and training (McNeill et al., 2012). Curricula and programmes in undergraduate midwifery already contain substantial public health teaching and learning, but inclusive approaches around midwives using approaches and principles of communication such as brief intervention and motivational interviewing are not standardised and are often seen as skills for specialists or for midwives who work in particular roles or areas of practice.

# Public Health and Midwifery
## DEFINITIONS AND LANGUAGE
Public health as a concept has existed since the 19th century. The idea behind it is that raising the health and wellbeing of individuals or groups has a positive impact on the whole of society. Initially public health was focused on public works, which had an impact on whole groups—clean drinking water, good sewerage or safe food, for example (Berridge et al., 2011). By the early 20th century public health initiatives were much more targeted. Mothers and babies were a particular focus of interventions as they were seen to be the future of society. Infant welfare clinics were developed alongside health visitors. As part of this targeted public health drive the 1902 Midwives Act was passed which made midwifery a legally protected profession with its own training and regulations (McIntosh, 2012). This reminds us that public health and midwifery have always been linked. In contemporary practice the work of the midwife is focused on individual public health support and interventions, which in turn benefits all society. Smoking cessation support, for example, has a clear impact on the physical health of the individual as well as other members of the family including babies and children. More broadly it also benefits society by reducing poor respiratory health and cancer and negative impacts on the NHS.

Moreover, there are some areas of midwifery which are instantly recognised as having a direct contribution to the public health agenda, for example, diet and nutrition, perinatal screening, smoking and breastfeeding. Other areas such as physiological birth, safeguarding and domestic abuse are an important part of the midwifery public health agenda but do not always fit as comfortably or easily under the public health umbrella. There is a huge breadth and complexity in midwifery of public health opportunities and issues, which have the potential to make a difference to outcomes—and that all starts with the fundamentals of public health communication. Fig. 7.3 shows some of the elements of public health within midwifery, and which ones may seem more clearly part of the broad public health agenda and which ones less so.

However, without tailored communication knowledge and skills, public health messages are at risk of being ignored, diluted or ineffective. The building blocks

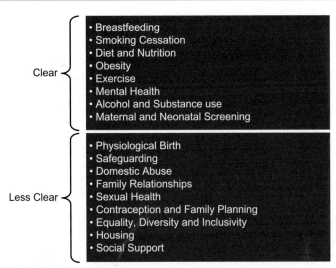

**Fig. 7.3** Public health within midwifery.

in facilitating excellence in public health communication include clarity around definitions, the use of clear language and terminology and forming meaning and understanding of public health issues. These building blocks are the basis of authentic conversations in public health, which impact other associated factors such as informed consent, information giving and evidence-based practice.

**QUICK REFLECTION**

Smoking 'cessation':
- Does this word often get confused with something else, e.g., 'sensation' or 'station'?
- Do people often ask what this word means?
- Do you use alternative definitions to aid understanding and clarity?

As we have seen in Chapter 3, midwifery has its own definitions and language which is not always clear to those who are either not immersed in it or working in maternity services. This can make it more difficult to facilitate and develop clarity and transparency in communication and sometimes may cause misunderstanding, offence or distress to families in our care.

We need to put ourselves in the position of the families that we care for to get across effective public health communication. This includes thinking about how terms and language can be simplified as appropriate, to convey the correct message and information needed to underpin informed decision-making. It is good practice to check back what has been discussed and that there is a mutual understanding if any decisions have been taken, what these are and what actions will arise from the conversation.

## FIRST 1000 DAYS

A crucial and underpinning concept of the midwifery contribution to public health is the concept of the 'first 1000 days' (House of Commons: Health and Social Care Committee, 2019). This is an evidence-based focus which supports a concentration of knowledge, resources and actions spanning from the time of conception to the child's age of 2 years (24 months) (Darling et al., 2020). The approach of the first 1000 days is considered essential and integral to many aspects of public health, and as midwives we have an enormous part to play in the window of opportunity that childbearing offers (Darling et al., 2020).

Making a difference to outcomes in maternal and child health is reliant upon many broad influencing factors, and these are essentially built upon positive and authentic approaches to communication. Understanding the importance of the first 1000 days, and how our individual roles and responsibilities within the delivery of maternity services can contribute, is the first step in thinking more deeply about why and how midwives make a real difference to families' lives (Darling et al., 2020).

## UNIVERSAL CARE AND THOSE WITH ADDITIONAL NEEDS

One of the most significant pieces of research to explore the breadth and depth of the impact that midwives have on the health of women, babies and families was published in *The Lancet* (Renfrew et al., 2014). The concept and notion of universal care and care for women with additional needs was clearly set out and discussed. It outlines a framework for delivery of care across a spectrum of needs throughout the childbearing continuum, with particular relevance to public health and improving outcomes (Renfrew et al., 2014). The notion of a universal care approach has been around for a number of years, from the birth of Sure Start and Children's Centres in the early 2000s to Marmot identifying the importance of this in 2010, but it wasn't until *The Lancet* series that the approach was highlighted as the path going forward and main driver in public health maternity care (Renfrew et al., 2014).

The idea is that midwives use core communication skills when delivering public health information, messages and interventions as part of universal care, then draw on their specialist skills for more complex factors when caring for those with additional needs. This ensures that an empathic person-centred holistic communication is front and centre when utilising a wide range of midwifery knowledge and skills (Crabbe & Hemingway, 2014). The training and knowledge midwives build during their careers provide a good foundation for further development of skills in communication around public health issues. A key message is for us to use these as the building blocks to make connections and establish positive and meaningful relationships with those families in our care.

Midwives are already carrying many of the key communication tools in our kit-bags of care that we can use as a starting point when thinking about pathways for care and how to embed public health approaches. Fig. 7.4 illustrates the main elements of this kitbag, which are vital in all situations.

It is not enough, however, to carry these communication tools in our midwifery kitbags if we never get them out and use them, or we do not use them correctly. We also need to make sure that we regularly 'clean out' our kitbags and see what tools need renewing or replacing, and if we need to add in any new tools, which would improve our communication approach. There are also tools in our kitbags that we are perhaps more skilled at using, and others in which we need further education, training or practice. Effective communication is also flexible; we use different elements in different ways in the communication differently depending on what elements of public health we are delivering and to whom.

## COFFEE BREAK ACTIVITY

- Make a note of your personal kitbag communication tools.
- What tools would you like to add to your own kitbag?
- Are there any tools which you would leave to one side?

One element of the kitbag which we may not be so familiar with is the call to 'follow the narrative'. As midwives we, and the families that we care for, are shaped by the stories that make us who we are, how we behave and how we make sense of ourselves in the context of our lives. These multiple stories and experiences are reflected in our morals, beliefs and values and together they weave the narratives of our life course (Frank, 2010). The families that we look after all have different, unique and distinct narratives, their lives lived in the context of many different factors which are played out in our communications and lifestyles. It is this ability to find, understand and be guided by others' narratives that is key in successful midwifery public health communications. As midwives we need to start with the mindset of knowing those whom we care for, and why they make the decisions and choices that they do, listening and respecting the reasoning, which is shared in the stories that they share with us. If we do this then we can be confident in our approach to starting a healthy conversation around public health issues.

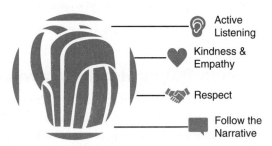

**Fig. 7.4**   The midwife's communication kitbag.

**QUICK REFLECTION**

Think about how to start healthy conversations:
- What does our communication look like to others?
- Why do we use the communication tools that we do?

## HEALTH PROMOTION AND LIFESTYLE CHOICES

*Public health* is concerned with the broad social good. *Health promotion* is a vital element of public health which is targeted at individuals. Most of the public health work that midwives do is based around health promotion. Health promotion in midwifery is often seen as the preserve of prenatal and antenatal care, but it is important throughout the whole of the childbearing continuum. There are multiple opportunities as a midwife to encourage and discuss a range of issues to promote a healthier lifestyle, which can have beneficial impacts for women, babies and families (Marshall et al., 2019).

To return to the example of smoking, discussions around reducing and quitting smoking, second-hand smoke, passive smoking and smoke-free homes, plus healthy houses (environments) are all part of public health initiatives to reduce disease, improve perinatal short- and long-term outcomes and help with financial control for those in smoking households/environments. The evidence regarding disease prevention in mother and baby is clear, and there is a package of methods that midwives now use as part of care and communications around smoking in the childbearing continuum for the family (Renfrew et al., 2014).

**PRACTICE POINTS**
- Prior to starting the conversation, read the history.
- Have information on support, referrals and care pathways to hand.
- Individual, holistic and person-centred care is key.
- An empathetic, nonjudgemental approach goes a long way.
- Comprehensive 'fact checking'—getting it right first time.
- Checking back with the family in your care—the right details.
- Embedding discussion around the 'Who, Why, Where and How' of information sharing—an essential part of care.
- Paying attention to terminology and use of language.
- Ensure sufficient time for discussions.

# Communication in Public Health Midwifery

To understand the importance of communication in public health midwifery, it is essential to reflect on the role of the midwife in public health, and how this is essential across the whole of the childbearing continuum. We have considered the complexities of communicating public health agendas and strategies and the need that midwives can have for support and training in this area. Difficulties can arise in the one-size-fits-all nature of some public health advice and the need to balance this with a trust-building individualised approach. For example, it has been known since the early 1960s that smoking has negative impacts on both adult and foetus. The message that smoking is bad therefore seems simple and uncontroversial. However, to say this to women and pregnant people who are smoking risks being seen as patronising and demeaning. In order to give effective support, we need to listen and to understand individual drivers and perspectives. Women will usually know the negative effects of smoking, but for them the positive psychological impacts of the habit may outweigh these. We need to come alongside women and build meaningful relationships in order that public health interventions can have a chance of being effective.

---

### Case Study

#### Smoking in Pregnancy

Consider the scenario:

Sara is a G3 P2 and is 28 weeks pregnant. She booked for care at 16 weeks, and she tells you that she smokes between 10 and 15 cigarettes per day since she was 16 years old. Sara smoked throughout both her last pregnancies and struggled to quit. She has a difficult relationship with her partner, and they currently do not live together. Sara is new to the area having just moved in, feels quite isolated from her family and missed her last midwife appointment. She enjoys smoking as some time to herself, to take a break and to relieve stress. She attends her 28-week appointment at the GP with her children but had to get two buses and is worried about the cost of the fare.

- Thinking about the public health aspect of midwifery care in this scenario, can you identify any additional needs that Sara and her family may have, and how you can provide information, guidance and support?
- As Sara's midwife what will your communication approach be when discussing smoking in pregnancy?
- What aspects of this scenario are important influencing factors in tailoring communication to Sara and her family needs?

---

## HOW TO APPROACH PUBLIC HEALTH COMMUNICATION

Reflecting on the foregoing scenario, we can see that midwives have a unique position in women's and families' lives at this time, to be enablers and providers of public health care. Delivering excellence in communication for public health issues relies on the following important factors:

- Creating a central focus on **building a relationship** with the woman, birthing person and family/friends.
- Using this focus to develop an **understanding of needs** and wishes.
- Incorporate as your baseline a **nonjudgemental** approach.
- Using the **triennium of strands** of evidence-based practice, midwifery knowledge and experience and instinct to inform and support decision-making.

Effective and successful use of these factors, as outlined earlier, will enable you as a midwife to develop a personal approach to communication, applicable to a wide range of public health situations and scenarios.

This building on and around approach, much like a jigsaw (Marshall et al., 2019), acts as a starting point, wherever you are in your midwifery career, from thinking about applying to study midwifery, through training as a student and to practising as a newly qualified midwife and beyond.

**QUICK REFLECTION**

Think about a scenario when you were involved with public health communication or use the case study provided earlier.
- Reflect on your approach—why you took this path, and how the communication determines or influences outcomes.
- Can you develop, incorporate or improve on the communication style/s that you used to become more empathic and meaningful?
- How could this be led by the woman/birthing person?

Ideas about the delivery of public health messages can often be quite old-fashioned and paternalistic. Information is given to women or birthing people who passively receive, absorb and act on it. In reality all effective relationships require flexibility and negotiation. As midwives we should explore the options of shared or co-participation/creation and recognition of the issues that are important for individuals. As part of this, we need to consider the notion of power balance/imbalance between midwife and mother, before we can seek to develop and improve public health communication with families whom we care for. We are often seen as the 'expert' and our knowledge and information more important than the people we are communicating with. It is up to us to come alongside people and work to break down the barriers that the imbalance in power can throw up.

We can do this by taking our lead from the woman/birthing person, developing a co-communication approach to public health in maternity, in which the direction is led and decided by women/birthing people, not by midwives and maternity services. We can also look to ourselves and raise awareness of how different communication approaches may impact factors such as relationship building, which are key in public health maternity care. One way of doing this is to be reflexive and think about and acknowledge how our position and role as a caregiver in maternity influence our approach to communicating public health. Secondly, we can use reflection to help us improve and understand different styles and ways of communicating. Being a reflexive and reflective midwife will enable you to challenge your current approach and identify where improvements can be made, and where additions may be needed—we go back to our *midwives kitbag* (Fig. 7.4) to guide us. By doing this we foster positive actions which can lead to supporting our personal development through enhancing communication skills, building on the need to be dynamic, flexible and ready to embrace change.

Supporting co-communication can be a challenge because of the way NHS maternity services are currently funded, designed, organised and delivered, even with service user input. This approach to care can be more commonly seen and experienced through other providers such as private and independent midwifery services. However, organisational support through personalised midwifery schemes in the NHS including meaningful continuity of care will hopefully allow for co-communication to develop.

## PRACTICE POINTS

Communicating *with* people not *at* them:
- Self-awareness of personal boundaries and needs, and how this can affect communication.
- Sensitivity and ability to identify potential challenging areas or topics and adjust as needed.
- To work towards co-communication.
- Acknowledge the importance of decision-making as the woman/birthing person's inherent right.

As midwives we are often deemed to be facilitators of care and decision-making, which may be true in some circumstances, but we need to move away from the notion of shared decision-making and towards the notion of individual decision-making. It is important to recognise and appreciate that women/birthing people are more than capable of making their own decisions around public health issues, and we as their caregivers should be equally capable of understanding and respecting this as a valid and effective approach.

There is such a breadth and depth of public health issues to be navigated and considered during the childbearing continuum that should be informed and directed by the woman/birthing person—as to what is important to them, not what we as midwives consider to be important.

If we refer back to the case study (smoking in pregnancy), we can consider this in a different way. Although as midwives we may have a duty of care to discuss smoking in the antenatal period as the primary public health concern, this may not be what the woman/birthing person thinks or wants. Think again about Sara's situation, and when you approach communication how this may need to be adapted or changed—if Sara's main concern is family relationships, financial or transport issues and not smoking then you need to flex your communication towards Sara's identified needs.

In the next section we will consider how we support and encourage women/birthing people with their identified needs and wishes to change, through public health communication approaches and use of select methods.

# Considering Actions, Understanding the Situation, Working in Context

A crucial element of public health communication in midwifery is a working knowledge of decision-making and public health behaviours in communities, and how as midwives we can support change through informed and empowering conversations. This can be seen as a basic three-step process which can be applied to a broad range of public health issues within maternity (Fig. 7.5).

Let's look at the **first step** in the process, *considering actions*. Before we do anything, we need to consider the lifestyle choices and behaviours of those families that we care for. This involves looking at and discussing those choices as appropriate, which will help us to gain an overall view and think about any influencing factors which impact and influence those choices and actions. This first step will help us to assess and review individual needs on a holistic basis, so we can gain a comprehensive understanding of the current situation and why this might impact on a person's public health choices. This information leads to our **second step**, which is *understanding the situation*. The assessment and review will vary according to the public health area being looked at, and various tools (for example, care pathways) are available to help with this element of the process.

Moving on, the **third step** allows us to consider the *context* in which we are practising as midwives and the context in which the families live their lives and how this influences choices and actions. As midwives we work and practise in a range of varied roles and environments, which incorporate differing degrees and elements of the maternity public health agenda. For example, a core midwife working on a labour ward will have different perspectives to a continuity of care midwife, or an independent midwife. All will have some elements of public health within their midwifery role, but these will vary in nature, depth and breadth according to how and where they practise.

The *context* of family life is an important one, and this is impacted by the varied nature and structure of the families that we care for. Context can only be understood when a respectful relationship is developed between the midwife and woman/birthing person, as context is not just about what we observe, but the meaning that

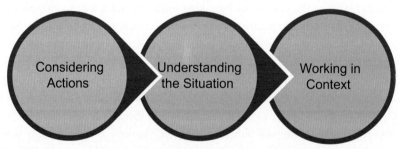

**Fig. 7.5** Three-step communication approach to support change in maternity public health issues.

this has for others, and this needs to be understood and acknowledged as an important aspect of communication. Only then can we fully appreciate person behaviours and choices and support those who wish to work towards change.

With this stepped process we can also identify any constraints which may make impactful and successful public health communication difficult or challenging, and we are going to consider this aspect next through reflection.

---

**COFFEE BREAK ACTIVITY**

Consider how to work within constraints and deal with barriers in public health communication:
- Think about your current midwifery role, where you work, the environment, the nature of the care you deliver—in essence the context of where you work—and list the three most important/biggest elements.
- How do these elements have the potential to limit your ability in public health communications?
- Identify barriers within these limitations, then consider potential actions which may help to reduce or remove these.

---

It is important that we identify and tackle perceived, potential and actual barriers in the context of where we work and how we work, as these are essential in being able to select and communicate appropriate and individualised information and offering any further support such as brief intervention.

Prior to implementing further input such as brief intervention, research has suggested that midwives have identified a number of barriers around delivering suitable public health communications to women/birthing people and families (Gomez & Chilvers, 2017; McNeill et al., 2012; Sanders et al., 2016). These were identified as lack of confidence in discussing sensitive subjects, lack of time and lack of multi-professional training (Gomez & Chilvers, 2017).

Training around public health communications appears to be focused on the information that midwives give, which is important, but can often have less attention on the approach and how the message is given. The steps, discussions and reflections in this chapter should help with this element, but education, training and knowledge in public health communication should aim to utilise scenarios, case studies and role play through experiential learning, alongside the facts and figures of information giving.

# Targeted Approaches to Public Health Communication

## BRIEF INTERVENTION TRAINING

The World Health Organization (WHO) defines brief interventions as 'practices that aim to identify a real or potential alcohol (or other drug) problem and motivate an individual to do something about it' (WHO, 2018). Despite this targeted definition, the technique of brief intervention is increasingly used across a range of public health issues. In essence it is facilitating very short, focused conversations designed to support change around health behaviours. It has been used in midwifery largely in the areas of smoking cessation, alcohol intake and dietary intake. Clearly the idea is suitable for some areas/topics more than others—for sensitive issues additional time may be needed and this approach may not be suitable. The approach of brief intervention is based around the core of *information giving*; it is not about reciprocity or discussion which requires alternative in-depth methods. Research around the effectiveness of brief intervention is mixed (McNeill et al., 2012). However, targeted use as part of a toolkit of care is useful and it is often used alongside other tools or approaches such as screening, care pathways and referral to specialist services.

There are several different brief intervention models and approaches that can be utilised in practice by midwives, and those that seem to work best have communication skills at the heart of the teaching and learning approach. One such example of this is using an approach called 'Healthy Conversation Skills', in which midwives can utilise their contacts with women/birthing people and families, in an opportunistic way through practical communications methods to initiate brief intervention on certain topics (Lawrence et al., 2020).

This method develops skills that midwives already use such as reflection and listening, adds other skills such as goal setting, and uses the unique trust-built relationship that midwives have with families to confidently use healthy conversations in public health communications. The interventions are often opportunistic rather than planned and work best if specific and tailored information is offered.

## POINTS TO CONSIDER WHEN BRIEF INTERVENTION AND FURTHER INPUT MAY BE REQUIRED

- Additional time and/or appointments.
- Flexibility of schedule of contacts.
- Education and training needed to deliver appropriate approaches/models.
- Alignment with guidelines, policies and evidence-based practice.
- Use of other roles within the multidisciplinary team to deliver targeted public health maternity communications.
- Making use of referrals, specialist practitioners and services.
- Incorporating the use of motivational interviewing techniques.

## DYNAMIC NARRATIVES

Some of the most challenging elements of public health communication in midwifery occur when we care for those families who have several wide-ranging issues, which may impact behaviours and lifestyle resulting in poorer health outcomes.

There is an increasing recognition of the value that storytelling can play in building relationships and in constructing understanding (Saffran, 2021). For the public this may be through Mumsnet or Instagram, but storytelling can also be used in a therapeutic context to support individuals' public health goals. Women/birthing people's stories can provide the building blocks for co-communication and improved outcomes. Fig. 7.6 demonstrates the purpose and impact of storytelling in public health.

It is in these situations that understanding those families' individual stories, and how they are woven into the childbearing continuum, can help us as midwives to see and listen to the context of life stories. If we can do this, we can build on creating a path of co-communication with families and a more meaningful and positive public health journey. This can reveal the broader narratives that influence the decision-making of women and birthing people, and how these narratives can shift and change throughout childbearing.

If we think back to the case study that we considered earlier on, we can think about Sara's choices and how her life and decision-making are shaped by what is important to her in her life. When we build that relationship and co-communication with Sara we may find out that one important factor is Sara's relationship with her partner, and that the dynamics of this relationship are a significant influencing factor in the decisions that Sara makes. As Sara's midwife we need to build this knowledge into our public health communications and consider how this may affect health and wellbeing for Sara and her family. It is not unusual for smoking to be a

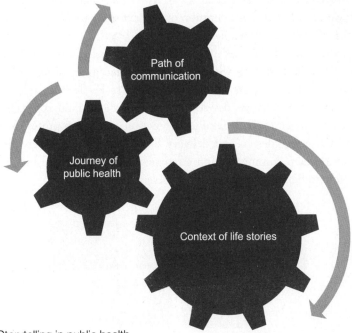

**Fig. 7.6** Storytelling in public health.

stress reliever and coping mechanism for women/birthing people, and for Sara, it may help her to cope with the difficulties in her partner relationship. With this in mind a different and tailored approach to discussing smoking in pregnancy will be needed, and alternative options discussed.

---

**COFFEE BREAK ACTIVITY**

Think about the different stories that you encounter which directly or indirectly are part of public health and are impacted by communications:
- How do you identify and encounter these stories?
- How do you take these into account in your co-communication?
- Why are these stories important?

---

For some people behaviour change around public health may be very challenging or even not appropriate at that point. This could be because there are other factors and issues in their life which are more important/take up time. If we understand their stories we will better understand what might or might not be possible in terms of change. Listening to stories will also help us to see lifestyle behaviours in context—they may be long established, complex and rooted in emotional and psychosocial factors (the life stories). Using dynamic narratives may allow us to come alongside people and mitigate the negative effects of an unequal power-based relationship which would normally put the professional 'in charge'.

When we consider the stories and narratives that make up the life course of maternity, we can see that consideration of context is an anchor point for communication, for example, as shown in Fig. 7.7.

The context in which families' life stories are governed and shaped is determined by a range of broader narratives which include economic and political policy-making and government decisions. As midwives we need to be flexible and adaptable as context and narratives change, developing a dynamic and fluid approach to public health co-communication with families. Sometimes as health professionals we are constrained by service design and delivery, but we need to think creatively about how we can develop communication strategies with women and birthing people which are able to flex with differing life-course pathways.

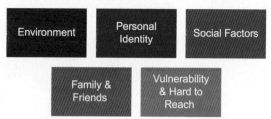

**Fig. 7.7**   Understanding context in public health communication.

# Conclusion

Communication in public health along the childbearing continuum can be a challenging road to navigate but is one which is essential in the offer of care and incorporation of co-communication. We have explored the principles of communication in public health and have considered a range of communication techniques and tools which midwives can use to deliver and develop their practice. Smoking cessation has been taken as the example topic, but the ideas and techniques are applicable and useful in all midwifery. We have considered the importance of stories and narratives in decision-making and how this can impact decision-making and life choices and influence public health behaviours in families. It is important that we reflect on our own knowledge, skills and attitudes and use communication to come alongside women and people in the childbearing year. Although we are tasked with delivering broad public health goals, we will be most successful if we see the people we are caring for holistically and as individuals rather than simply as problems or targets. Our communication should always be:

- Accessible to all
- Tailored and determined by the individual and family
- Be the best fit for the life course
- We listen, respect, trust and understand

---

**QUICK REFLECTION**

- What have you learnt about communication in public health as a midwife?
- Can you identify elements of communication in public health to improve or change in your own role and the environment in which you practice?
- How can you work towards a co-communication approach with the families that you care for?

---

## References

Acheson, D. (1988). *Public health in England: The report of the Committee of Inquiry Into the Future Development of the Public Health Function* (pp. 23–34). The Stationery Office.

Berridge, V., Gorksy, M., & Mold, A. (2011). *Public health in history.* Open University Press.

Crabbe, K., & Hemingway, A. (2014). Public health and wellbeing: A matter for the midwife? *British Journal of Midwifery, 22*(9), 634–640.

Darling, J. C., Bamidis, P. D., Burberry, J., & Rudolf, M. C. J. (2020). The First Thousand Days: Early, integrated and evidence-based approaches to improving child health: Coming to a population near you? *Archives of Disease in Childhood, 105,* 837–841.

Department of Health/Public Health England. (2013a). *The evidence base of the public health contribution of nurses and midwives.* Department of Health.

Frank, A. (2010). *Letting stories breathe: A socio-narratology.* University of Chicago Press.

Gomez, E., & Chilvers, R. (Eds.) for Royal College of Midwives (RCM) (2017). Stepping up to public health: A new maternity model for women and families, midwives and maternity support workers [online]. RCM. https://www.rcm.org.uk/media/3165/stepping-up-to-public-health.pdf. Accessed: 29 July 2021.

House of Commons: Health and Social Care Committee. (2019). *First 1000 days of life, thirteenth report of session 2017–19.* Parliamentary Copyright House of Commons.

Lawrence, W., Vogel, C., Strömmer, S., Morris, T., Treadgold, B., Watson, D., Hart, D., McGill, K., Hammond, J., Harvey, N. C., Cooper, C., Inskip, H., Baird, J., & Barker, M. (2020). How can we best use opportunities provided by routine maternity care to engage women in improving their diets and health? *Journal of Maternal and Child Nutrition, 16,* e12900.

Marshall, J., Baston, H., & Hall, J. (2019). *Midwifery essentials: Public health.* (Vol. 7). Elsevier.

McIntosh, (2012). *A social history of maternity care.* Routledge.

McNeill, J., Doran, J., Lynn, F., Anderson, G., & Alderdice, F. (2012). Public health education for midwives and midwifery students: A mixed methods study. *BMC Pregnancy Childbirth, 12,* 142.

Meegan, S. (2020). Revised standards of proficiencies for midwives: An opportunity to influence childhood health? *British Journal of Midwifery, 28*(3), 150–154.

Renfrew, M. J., McFadden, A., Bastos, M. H., Campbell, J., Channon, A. A., Cheung, N. F., Silva, D. R., Downe, S., Kennedy, H. P., Malata, A., McCormick, F., Wick, L., & Declercq, E. (2014). Midwifery and quality care: Findings from a new evidenced-informed framework for maternal and newborn care. *The Lancet, 384,* 1129–1145.

Saffran, L. (2021). Public health storytelling practice. *The Lancet, 397,* 1536–1537.

Sanders, J., Hunter, B., & Warren, L. (2016). A wall of information? Exploring the public health component of maternity care in England [online]. *Midwifery, 34,* 253–260.

## Further Reading and Resources

RCM: i-learn. https://www.rcm.org.uk/promoting/learning-careers/i-learn-and-i-folio/. Accessed 01 January 2022.

> *The Royal College of Midwives has collated a great set of resources for improving your learning, knowledge and skills around a wide range of public health issues in midwifery. You can access these through the RCM website if you are a member. They consist of interactive sessions in varying depths and offer short as well as longer more in-depth sessions. These can be a useful starting point in knowledge development or as refresher sessions.*

## Specific Websites

Leicestershire Government: Making Every Contact Count (MECC) (2020). Healthy conversation skills: Having healthy conversations website. https://www.healthyconversationskills.co.uk/. Accessed: 01 December 2022.

> *Although MECC has been around for a few years, the approach is a valid one, and this compact and easy-to-navigate website, supported by a number of Councils in the Leicestershire area, focuses on the model of healthy conversation skills. Information, advice and some online sessions are available to boost your baseline knowledge and skills.*

National Health Service (NHS) England. Maternity Transformation Programme. https://www.england.nhs.uk/mat-transformation/. Accessed: 01 January 2022 (Covering Local Maternity Systems (LMS).

> *This website uses videos, weblinks and information to give a comprehensive overview of the Maternity Transformation Programme (England), with reference to key maternity drivers, changes made and plans going forwards. Although not specifically about public health, it covers a number of public health issues in maternity.*

Nursing and Midwifery Council (NMC). Resources and templates for revalidation. https://www.nmc.org.uk/revalidation/resources/. Accessed: 01 January 2022.

> *A range of information is provided through this part of the NMC website, telling you what revalidation is, how to revalidate and providing all the forms and documents needed. There are interactive sessions and videos on revalidation and the different ways that professionals can achieve this three-yearly requirement for registration.*

Nursing and Midwifery Council (NMC). Standards for pre-registration midwifery programmes: Part 3 of Realising professionalism: Standards for education and training. https://www.nmc.org.uk/standards/standards-for-midwives/standards-for-pre-registration-midwifery-programmes/. Accessed: 01 January 2022.

*This section of the NMC website provides detailed documents on the current standards for pre-registration midwifery. This is useful reading as it outlines what is expected in terms of the public health learning and teaching in midwifery curricula and programmes, and how this feeds into the future midwife.*

Public Health England, replaced by UK Health Security Agency and Office for Health Improvement and Disparities. https://www.gov.uk/government/organisations/public-health-england

*This is the main website for Public Health England, which is often a good starting point for any public health or related information. Here you will find a range of useful documents, policies, guidelines and projects.*

Public Health England, Fingertips. Public health profiles: Child and maternal health. https://fingertips.phe.org.uk/profile/child-health-profiles

*For a specific focus on maternal and child health this section of the PHE website is the one to use as your baseline for information. You can look at current campaigns, projects and targets, and access useful information on trends in public health in maternity.*

Public Health England (2021). Healthy beginnings: Applying all our health. https://www.gov.uk/government/publications/healthy-beginnings-applying-all-our-health

*This section of the website is a mine of useful resources across public health, not specifically aimed at maternal and child health, but very useful when caring for families. The resources include opportunities for e-learning, interactive sessions and links to key reports and are based on the healthy beginnings report and how you can put this into practice as a health professional.*

Royal Society for Public Health (RSPH) website. https://www.rsph.org.uk/

United Nations Children's Fund (UNICEF) website. https://www.unicef.org.uk/

World Health Organization (WHO) website. https://www.euro.who.int/en/home

### Key/Seminal Texts

Acheson, D. (1988). *Public health in England: The report of the Committee of Inquiry into the Future Development of the Public Health Function* (pp. 23–34). The Stationery Office.

House of Commons: Health and Social Care Committee. (2019). *First 1000 days of life, thirteenth report of session 2017–19*. Parliamentary Copyright House of Commons.

Marmot, M. (2010). Fair society, healthy lives: The Marmot Review: Strategic review of health inequalities in England post-2010. Dept for International Development. https://www.gov.uk/research-for-development-outputs/fair-society-healthy-lives-the-marmot-review-strategic-review-of-health-inequalities-in-england-post-2010.

Renfrew, M. J., McFadden, A., Bastos, M. H., Campbell, J., Channon, A. A., Cheung, N. F., Silva, D. R., Downe, S., Kennedy, H. P., Malata, A., McCormick, F., Wick, L., & Declercq, E. (2014). Midwifery and quality care: Findings from a new evidenced-informed framework for maternal and newborn care. *The Lancet, 384*, 1129–1145.

# CHAPTER 8

# Communication and Complex Care Planning

Katie Christie ▪ Jane Cleary

As we have seen in previous chapters, society and communication are ever changing. Pregnant women and people are facing new challenges every day as they navigate their pregnancies. There are always medical advances as well as living and surviving in a demanding society that now is dominated by social media. Communication has changed and expectations of the birthing community have put the traditional NHS models of care under question. As a midwifery and obstetric profession, we need to identify that we are meeting the needs and expectations of our clientele and where our care and communication require development or reassessment. More importantly we need to understand our clients before we can really support them through their pregnancies.

**COFFEE BREAK ACTIVITY**

- Look at the section on 'complexity' in Chapter 5.
- How would you define 'complexity'?
- What do we need to remember when talking about 'complexity' with clients?

This chapter covers principles which are relevant to all people in all pregnancies—care, compassion, flexibility of approach and open and honest communication. However, it focuses on pregnancies and births which could be considered to be 'complex'. We have already considered the idea of 'complexity' in Chapter 5 and you may find it useful to revisit that section before embarking on this chapter.

Communication is one of the elements of complex care planning, but the most important one. This chapter will use real-world examples to explore some of the issues and challenges of planning and providing complex care. It begins by considering typical care pathways and ways we may need to adapt these to suit individual people. It then explores the importance of multidisciplinary communication before using case studies to explore examples of care. Every pregnancy is complex in its own way because the path it will take and the outcome are unknown. This means that the principles discussed in this chapter are relevant to all people throughout the childbearing year. However, the focus on complexity and supportive pathways through it offers you ideas to develop your own practice in this area.

## Limitations of Routine Antenatal Care

Antenatal care has existed in something very similar to its current form since the 1920s (McIntosh, 2012). Initially it was designed purely to pick up major physical issues in pregnancy such as pathologically high blood pressure. Over time it has evolved and both midwives and pregnant people now use it as a time to discuss a whole range of physical, emotional and psychological factors and to develop a professional relationship (see Chapter 3 for discussion of this). Professionals seek to provide individualised care, but time limits and checklists can have a significant negative impact on what can be achieved. Time is a massive factor. Take a community midwife, for example. They have 20–30 minutes per appointment to ensure that a woman and her baby remain safe throughout their pregnancy. For a low-risk pregnancy this might just be enough time to go through all their needs, for example, their medical wellbeing, urine and blood pressure testing and then consider their social wellbeing. What would this look like if a woman presented with previous birth or sexual trauma at her booking appointment?

**QUICK REFLECTION**

Think back to an antenatal clinic you have attended recently.
- How much time was there for each appointment?
- Did you feel you were able to answer any questions/concerns in appropriate detail?
- How would you have managed a complex conversation given the time limits?

In many organisations there are extra services to support women and the community midwife throughout the pregnancy, birth and the postnatal period. Understandably at times even this is not enough and relationships and the opportunities for women to really get the support they require can be missed. This risks any stress or trauma growing, and an issue that might have been relatively simple to tackle with the right support at the right time becomes more complex and significant. Evidence has suggested that continuity of care models (where a woman is cared for by a known midwife or team of midwives throughout the childbearing year) increase satisfaction and may reduce the impact of stress or trauma (NHS England, 2016). This is because women and people will have the same care provider throughout allowing relationships to form and therefore trust to develop. Women do not have to tell complex or traumatic stories over and over to different professionals, instead they can work with their midwife to build resilience and strategies for care and support. Many midwifery models have tried to incorporate the continuity theme within their care provisions particular for those with complex needs. However, this model does require commitment and investment on the part of teams and management. This has been hard to achieve under current conditions and has led to the Ockenden Report (Ockenden, 2022) calling for further implementation of continuity of care to be shelved until basic staffing levels are met in Trusts. Nevertheless, it remains an effective way to support women and families, particularly in cases with known complexities.

Regardless of the model of care we work through, it is our job as health professionals to work with clients to gain a full and accurate picture of their circumstances, expectations and needs during their pregnancy journey. It is so important to remember that every woman and person is unique. We see large numbers of pregnant women and people come through our services, and to manage this we must assume that women and people will generally present in similar ways throughout. The data we have about pregnancy and birth back this up and have led to the development of care schedules like antenatal care pathways. This is evidence based and of course will keep most women safe in their pregnancies. However, when we have women entering our services who have complex needs, we need to have the skills to manage their needs by listening, talking and escalating. We also need to be alert to the fact that women on standard pathways may develop additional psychological, social, medical or obstetric needs and that we need to be able to respond sensitively and appropriately.

Being pregnant can be a mixed experience for *all* pregnant women and people. Some would suggest that it is a very vulnerable time in their life. It is very much an unknown experience; even if it is a second, third or fourth pregnancy, it is always the first time for *this* pregnancy. Chapter 9 will explore how loss and trauma around pregnancy are individually defined and experienced. For some people issues such as infertility, previous miscarriage, emergency Caesarean section (C-section) instead of intended water birth, postnatal depression or lack of social support will leave them feeling anxious and vulnerable. Some women will have full trust in their own bodies, where some may have felt that their bodies have failed as they have either had miscarriages previously or gruelling rounds of in vitro fertilisation (IVF) treatment, for example. Some women and people may experience pregnancy as a loss of control and agency. Being told that their bodies have the capacity to grow a baby will not necessarily keep their anxieties at bay. These women will search for support from their care providers, so it is important that we meet their needs in order to engage them and to support foetal and maternal wellbeing throughout the pregnancy.

## Multidisciplinary Perspectives

As professionals working within a multidisciplinary environment, it is vital that we communicate effectively to best support women. As consultant midwives working with people with complex needs, we have had cases where after the time and hard work of developing engagement with a client, the relationship can be ruined in a second by another health professional who does not cater to their needs. This can be very common when so much of our conversations are guideline led rather than individualising the woman in relation to the guidance. This has led women and people to disengage altogether from the service and go alone. Women and people who are not getting the support they are searching for in their care providers or service will quite regularly feel that having no or limited care is safer for them and their baby.

Other chapters in this book have explored the importance of honest and effective communication between midwives and doctors and Chapter 3 considered the impact that different professional histories and philosophies have on communication. This has a significant impact on families and that the professional's behaviour lies at the heart of how women feel about their childbirth experience. Traditionally medicine has focused on the saving of life and has paid less attention to mental or emotional wellbeing. In situations where decisions must be made quickly this view can still prevail. The intention behind interventions is always an attempt to minimise the risk of poor or unfavourable outcomes. Chapter 5 noted the difficulties in judging risk and in talking about it.

Ultimately, we need to take care when we communicate with women and with each other. This means not falsely making complex decisions appear simple and not coercing women into making decisions they do not want to make, however well intentioned we may be. In the drive for physical safety we must never forget the need to support psychological wellbeing and to minimise the risk of harm emotionally. Through our communication—whether as doctors or midwives—we need to demonstrate that we value the need for a positive experience and that we understand that this matters to people. We need to be aware that our communication may make women feel less safe and in control and may back them into a corner. For example, they may choose a C-section over induction because they feel they will be more in control that way. Alternatively, they may feel pressured into choosing a vaginal birth when they want a C-section. Regardless of the situation or the ultimate decisions made, women must feel *listened to* and *heard*. Their caregiver must come alongside them and understand the many things that go to make up a situation, a feeling and a decision. Ultimately the woman who wanted a VBAC (vaginal birth after a Caesarean) may end up with a C-section but if she feels heard, supported and in control of what is happening and why, it is likely that trauma will be minimised, and wellbeing enhanced.

## Common Complex Care Planning Cases

The following sections explore in detail some of the complex scenarios which we may meet in practice. They are all individual and do not cover every challenging situation which you may experience. However, the principles of honest open and respectful communication are at the centre of each of these cases and are applicable anywhere and at any time.

**QUICK REFLECTION**

Think of an episode of complex care that you were involved in.
- What made it complex?
- Who was the lead caregiver?
- How was communication managed between the family and the multidisciplinary team?
- Do you feel that the communication was effective and appropriate?
- Could anything have been done differently to enhance communication?

## OUT OF GUIDELINE HOMEBIRTH

How we communicate is vital when we are ensuring that families are fully informed to give consent. As a midwife fundamentally we want women and their babies to have a safe outcome both physically and psychologically. Our role is to ensure clients are given the available information or evidence to make an informed choice. This needs to be presented in an unbiased format offering the alternatives alongside the risks and benefits.

The language and the way we share that information are relevant and will impact on the woman's decision or feelings about their individual choices. It can be challenging as the guidance and how it is published are not at times 'appropriate' for how we wish to share the information. For example, a discussion about the *chances* of situations happening compared to the *risk* of something occurring seems gentler and more accessible despite having the same meaning. An example of discussing 'risk', a very common conversation, is discussing the chances of a uterine rupture if planning a VBAC (the chances of it happening in labour is 1:200; RCOG, 2015). When women hear this, they will have mixed reactions. After all we have to remember that all people will assess risk differently because of individual factors, beliefs, previous experiences and so on. Some women see that as a high chance of uterine rupture happening and will not want to take the chance, whereas others will think that is a really low chance of it happening and do not feel worried about it at all. As the health professional it is hard to know that the woman you are informing has full insight into what you are discussing with them especially if they feel that there is a very low chance of a poor outcome. If uterine rupture occurs then it is clearly an obstetric emergency that needs to be managed in a timely manner to ensure that there is a positive outcome for the mother and the baby. Explaining this and the process of how we identify, respond and treat rupture can strengthen the importance of the information shared. When doing this, we need to remember to continue to treat women as individuals and to use language which is appropriate and comprehensible.

---

**Case Study**

**Complex Medical Conditions**

A community midwife contacted me after meeting with a woman and her partner when they were 28 weeks pregnant planning a homebirth, with numerous complications around the pregnancy. It was Louise's first baby, and with screening there was found to be a high chance of Down syndrome. Invasive testing was completed, and Trisomy 21 was confirmed. Group B strep had been detected in the pregnancy too. Louise engaged with the obstetric team but was clear with her community midwife that she would always plan a homebirth, and now with these added complications, this would not sway her decision, as long as she felt that her baby was not being compromised and she felt it would be safer to birth her baby in hospital. When speaking with the community midwife, I got the sense that this was a complex pregnancy that could potentially take a course that would involve early delivery. There were also signs that the baby was small for gestational age.

- *What do you feel are the key communication issues in this case study?*

---

## COMPLEX MEDICAL CONDITIONS

The MBRRACE report (MBRRACE-UK, 2021) is a yearly review of maternal deaths in the UK. One of its main aims is to look at how these deaths could have occurred and what we can learn from them to minimise future occurrences. One of the biggest recurring themes from the reports is the lack of communication between care providers and the pregnant woman or person. Very often we hear of women with medical needs in their pregnancies needing admission to the hospital to treat those medical needs and the admission not being shared to the appropriate teams for review. The simple task of sharing information between teams and different disciplines means that women will receive a full holistic review and an appropriate care plan. Take, for example, complex care planning for a woman who has a known cardiac condition. Before pregnancy she would have an allocated cardiologist to manage her condition. Once pregnant, the woman should be referred to an obstetrician, an anaesthetist and either her previous cardiologist or a maternal cardiologist specialist so that a care plan for her pregnancy management as well as the birth can be finalised. At times this is managed separately between the specialists. This involves a lot of appointments for the pregnant woman but also information can be lost in translation via letters between the specialists. From the data (Department of Health, 2013) we know that having all those specialists in one room during care planning allows the conversations to be concurrent. Questions and challenges can be presented immediately in a professional manner as the pregnant woman is also present. It allows the pregnant woman or person to be part of the process, ask questions directly and let them be the centre of the care planning process. This type of communication has directly improved women's and people's experiences of their pregnancy and birth. It humanises the care providers, allows women to know everything they need to know about their body and their baby and most importantly they feel like they are the ones in control.

Our team did not meet with Louise until she was 39 weeks pregnant. Up to that point she had continued to receive care from her community midwife, who in turn received support from the consultant midwives at the Trust. Louise believed in alternative therapies and natural remedies rather than turning to medication. Louise trusted her body and didn't require support from the hospital or the obstetric team, although she was happy with midwifery input as she felt that midwives supported 'normality'. However, there were aspects of care pathways and language used that Louise found very challenging. For example, with the Trisomy 21 diagnosis, she felt discriminated against for having a baby with Down syndrome as the service used this as a 'risk' factor and a reason for not birthing at home. Louise did not see this as a risk factor and felt well read in that a lot of babies with Down syndrome can birth normally and have well postnatal periods with some added support around feeding, but not much more than that. After quite a few appointments between 36 and 39 weeks, Louise withdrew from the service and felt quite pressured by every health professional she saw as induction of labour was recommended at each appointment. Louise only attended the appointments she felt would guide her in the information she needed to decide where would be the safest to birth, which were the foetal medicine scans. I eventually met with Louise after her last scan at 39 weeks, as I felt that I needed to have a frank conversation with her around risk versus benefits with the final scan review, putting a birth plan in place, and escalating this very complex homebirth to the full maternity team so that staff were supported in this situation. The local ambulance service was made aware as well as the neonatal team. An on-call homebirth team was put in place so that senior midwives would also be in attendance.

I spoke to Louise on the phone, and she was happy to discuss with me her final plans. It was important to her that I was not to discuss the risks as she clearly had heard it all from the multidisciplinary team and needed me instead to support her in her choices of giving birth at home. Louise was also considering freebirthing if we did not attend but would prefer a midwife with her as that felt safer to her. I agreed that after speaking about her pregnancy she was aware of the risks, and I too said that I needed to be clear with her before we proceed in the care planning, that I agreed with my colleagues and recommended induction of labour and birthing in the hospital setting so that we could have immediate neonatal support.

We both listened and respected each other's views and moved on. A care plan was agreed on, and the conversation felt positive. That same day Louise went on to labour and birthed her baby at home as she planned with midwifery support.

---

### Reflection on Case Study

- What key communication principles do you feel that this case study demonstrates?
- How do you think the quality of communication between the midwives and Louise impacted on her pregnancy and birth?

---

## BIRTH TRAUMA

Many of the complex care planning referrals that we receive as consultant midwives are from women expressing to their midwife feelings of trauma from their previous birth and an extreme fear in this pregnancy. At present around 30,000 women a year are reporting birth trauma from their birthing journeys in the UK (Birth Trauma Association, 2022). This may not mean that they have reached the full diagnostic criteria of post-traumatic stress disorder (PTSD) but they would describe their birth experience as traumatic. Beck (2004) has suggested that birth experience is 'in the eye of the beholder' or from their perception has feelings associated with trauma such as 'fear, helplessness, loss of control and horror'. For a detailed discussion of importance of seeing and communicating birth trauma as an individual experience, see Chapter 9.

Care planning for women who have experienced trauma can be challenging as they have often lost trust in the system and staff that work within it. Building relationships, listening and supporting open and honest communication are essential but still may not rebuild the bridges lost. Spending time understanding and acknowledging their story or perception of their experience in a supportive non-judgemental discussion is critical to ensure they feel heard. Making sense of what happened to them and not defending but sharing the care provider's perception alongside the competing pressures of the system can be helpful.

It is crucial when planning their care to consider how we can support families within the maternity services so they can feel safe and supported. Women will need to understand the risks and benefits of their individual decisions based on what these are alongside any existing medical or obstetric history so they can take responsibility and make an informed decision. Consideration of their emotional wellbeing needs to be at the centre of the discussion and recognition that this is as significant within their choices and plan. Through relationships and mutual trust we can empower women to make decisions that are safe for them and their baby both physically and emotionally if we recognise that they both have valued importance.

Kirkham (2010) discusses the often-narrow professional definition of safety, which essentially refers to a live mother and baby at the end of a defined period of care. However, women have a much wider and more subjective view of safety because as Edwards (2005) suggests, what makes them feel safe and cared for is the quality of the central relationship. Women need to be safe but, more essentially, they need to feel safe which is the responsibility of us as caregivers.

## Case Study

### Birth Trauma

Annemarie was referred to us early in her pregnancy. She was having care under a specialist maternal medicine team of midwives within the Trust's continuity of care model. It was evident that she had been seen predominantly by the same midwife and had received excellent continuity. On my initial meeting alongside the community midwife, it appeared that their relationship had been established. Annemarie seemed engaged, open and trusting in the meeting. She was receptive to my involvement which had been recognised due to her shared plans and choices which were out of hospital guidelines. Annemarie was 31 years old in her fourth pregnancy. She had a body mass index (BMI) of >45 at booking and had been diagnosed with gestational diabetes requiring insulin management. She had a history of depression and anxiety. She planned and hoped to have a vaginal birth in this pregnancy at home. Her past obstetric history had been x three lower segment Caesarean sections (LSCSs). In her first pregnancy she had a raised BMI of >50 and had a relatively normal pregnancy. She planned a vaginal birth, labouring spontaneously at 41 weeks' gestation. Due to delay in labour she had an epidural/augmentation and had an emergency LSCS of a large-for-dates (LFD) baby, 4763 kg. She had x two elective LSCSs at 38 weeks' gestation of LFD babies.

- *What do you feel are the key communication issues in this case study?*

On meeting Annemarie effective communication and listening to her perception of her previous birth experiences were felt to be the priority. It was evident that she was making decisions and choices that appeared unaligned with the perceived risk from an obstetric perspective. Making sense of her experience, acknowledging it and working collaboratively with Annemarie became the focus. It was apparent early in our meeting that she was still suffering with trauma symptoms from all of her previous experiences. Her particular focus was on the first pregnancy where she did not felt listened to or in control of any decisions and at times coerced into making decisions that she did not agree with. She was left with symptoms of trauma such as flashbacks, high levels of negative emotion and hypervigilance. At her subsequent births she felt that her experiences were similar in a system that did not support her. She felt coerced or bullied into having an elective LSCS without being listened to or respected. Annemarie expressed that throughout all of her pregnancies and births she had not been treated with respect or kindness and had often felt judged due to her size, social background and position as a woman in a misogynistic system.

Her mental health had never recovered following some treatment and support from perinatal services.

In her fourth pregnancy she had decided to take back control. She positioned herself with a vast amount of knowledge and research about her own history to enable her to fight for her human right to choose her decision declining obstetric involvement. It was clear that her trust, confidence and understanding of the system were severely damaged and it would take some time to rebuild this.

The priority within our communication was to establish mutual respect and understanding so we were able to rebuild the trust that had been so severely broken. Relationships and caring are grounded on universal humanistic values such as kindness, empathy and concern for others (Watson, 2009) and this was fundamental in our meetings. This took time and some meetings before we were able to start to consider her plan, choices and the safest options for Annemarie both physically and psychologically.

She declined to meet with the obstetric team initially for fear of being bullied and not listened to again. We spent time discussing her individual complexities and we used evidence that was available to have open conversations about the reason that obstetric care was recommended. She did agree to attend a meeting with an obstetrician, and we acted as her advocate in these meetings so she felt safe and heard.

Her diabetic conditions deteriorated in the last trimester of the pregnancy and there were increasing concerns about her placenta function as she passed her due date. She did not start labour spontaneously and at 42 weeks following discussion Annemarie decided to have an LSCS. She was able to articulate that she felt empowered to make that decision with shared knowledge and understanding. The experience was both positive and restorative for her mental wellbeing as she felt safe and in control of her own choice and decision. Although she was disappointed to not have the homebirth or vaginal birth that she so wished, being understood with respect, kindness and being in control made it a fulfilling experience without trauma or harm.

## PRACTICE POINTS

- Open respectful communication is fundamental in complex cases.
- Developing a trusting relationship with pregnant people and families can mean that their experience is positive even if the outcome is not as planned.
- Feeling empowered and in control can be vital to a positive experience for women and families.
- Honest communication does not mean hiding from uncomfortable conversations.

## FREEBIRTHING/UNASSISTED BIRTH

Freebirthing or unassisted birth is when a pregnant woman or person chooses to birth alone without a midwife or obstetrician present at the birth (Feeley & Thomson, 2016). It is legal in the UK. Unassisted birth in the UK appears to be rising and these have become an increasing number of our complex caseload. There are many reasons for this happening which are all very personal to individual families and each have their own complexities.

Any communication is fundamental for these women and people to ensure their safety throughout the pregnancy, birth and postnatal period. Listening, understanding and supporting them in their choices and decisions while sensitively sharing and documenting the potential risks are essential. As a midwife this may be both challenging and rewarding. Making sense of choices that do not fit with our personal model of care or perceived risk can be difficult and being without judgement our own values or beliefs. Coercive language or behaviour is often perceived as bullying and this needs to be avoided recognising their mental capacity to make the best decision for both them and their baby. We have to remember that in the main we all wish for the same outcome, that is, a healthy parent and baby. This includes mental and emotional health as well as physical health.

Previous birth trauma is often a theme that emerges with women choosing to opt out of the system and either limit the amount of access or only engage with specific care givers/periods. Occasionally they have had such a poor previous experience that when they are pregnant again they will decide that they will not engage at all and these are a group that we have limited data on.

The COVID-19 pandemic has impacted on this group of families and women chose to birth at home out of guidance to have their partner present (Greenfield et al., 2021). During the pandemic the homebirth service was suspended in many areas in the UK and many countries witnessed a rise in unassisted births. Birthing women and people were turning their backs on the maternity service because in their eyes, it was safer to birth at home and at times without a midwife. We have always had a proportion of the population that will freebirth, but because of what women were seeing in the press and on social media they were being terrified into thinking that a high-risk homebirth or freebirth was the safer option for them. We also have to remember that the vast majority of women who give birth will always choose what is safest for them and their baby and never purposely put themselves and their baby at harm.

Reaching out to pregnant women and people via social media platforms has massively improved how we access that group of the population. We are very aware that the majority of the population use social media to communicate, so we needed to have an understanding of their world. Regular positive images as well as current and real data around our local COVID-19 guidance meant that it was relevant to our clientele group and they could then relate as well as giving them a chance to contact us if they needed further support. In some cases, where we were really worried about certain women and people birthing at home, purely because they understandably needed their partners there throughout (at times when access to hospital for partners was severely restricted), it meant we could reach out and make robust plans for them on an individual basis when they entered the hospital environment.

## Case Study

### Freebirthing/Unassisted Birth

I was made aware of Jenny in my role as consultant midwife early on her pregnancy. The community midwife explained that Jenny planned to freebirth but would engage antenatally and postnatally in a limited way. This included no screening by ultrasound scan or blood tests. Jenny was happy to be palpated, have blood pressure checks, anything that was noninvasive. This also included only listening in to the foetal heart by pinard.

  • *What do you feel are the key communication issues in this case study?*

The community midwife led the care with my support. We agreed that nearer to the time of birth, I would offer to meet with Jenny and her partner to discuss the risks versus the benefits of freebirthing. After all, there can be so many different changes in pregnancy, which impacts on the woman changing how she views or manages her pregnancy and birth. It was also really important that the community midwife developed a good relationship with Jenny as much as possible because Jenny might decide she felt comfortable to have midwives present at her birth.

By 34 weeks of pregnancy Jenny remained certain that she was not having any scans. The community midwife and I decided it was a good time to meet Jenny together, which Jenny was happy with. Jenny was 36 weeks pregnant at the time we met her and her husband.

At first Jenny and her husband Steve seemed quite wary of me. My colleague had done her best to explain the reason why I was there, but I could tell that both were being cautious with me. After explaining who I was and my role, I always ask about the reasons they are choosing to birth out of guidance. I do this by explaining that it's important I understand their choices so that birth planning with them is more individualised. I also find it fascinating to hear why so many women do want to birth out of guidance. Jenny explained that it was her culture from her country of birth for women to birth with family and friends for support. Jenny also trusted her body and her baby that she could do this with no support from midwives. She had lacked trust in the maternity services in the UK.

Knowing where Jenny was coming from, it was clear she had good capacity and very much knew what was right for her. I thanked her for sharing the information with me, and explained that I understood, but would always want to advocate any woman having a midwife attend their birth for safety. It is always important that conversations with women in these situations are honest in both directions; we owe it to families to be honest and not to skirt around risks and challenges.

We then went over preparations for the birth. Jenny and Steve had clearly done their homework and watched a lot of footage around birth so felt confident that they could support their baby being born into water at home. We discussed the main emergencies that required immediate treatment, for example, neonatal resus and postpartum haemorrhage and how to contact help.

At T+17, Jenny gave birth, and with no signs of life at the time of birth, Jenny and Steve called an ambulance to assist. Jenny and Steve had not told anyone that Jenny was in labour, but from discussing it with them, the labour was average in length with the baby being birthed as Jenny planned for. When meeting with Jenny and Steve after the event they were very clear that they took full responsibility for the death of their child. No investigations were done on their request, as they felt that their choices had been met.

---

**PRACTICE POINTS**

- The person birthing the baby should be in control of decision-making with support from caregivers.
- Channels of communication should always be kept open—people and circumstances might change.
- Caring for, and communicating with, people who make different decisions from the ones we would make can be challenging.
- As practitioners we should use support structures and the wider multidisciplinary team to support us in giving care and debriefing after complex scenarios.

---

## Conclusion

This chapter has used a variety of case studies to illustrate how we communicate in complex scenarios and the impact that this can have on people and families. The principles of open, honest and respectful communication are always relevant, but for those with challenging circumstances the need to *listen* as well as *speak* is even more significant. For families in many of these cases, the need to be heard and validated within the system meant that the outcomes had meaningfully positive elements despite sometimes difficult outcomes.

There are challenges to midwives and other health care professionals in providing care in these circumstances—we have to juggle our own beliefs and feelings with those of our clients and with the expectations of the service. Self-awareness and support are essential to midwifery practice in these situations. Above all the willingness to develop a broad range of effective communication skills will support us in developing trusting relationships however complex the situation.

## References

Beck, C.T. (2004). Birth trauma: In the eye of the beholder, *Nursing Research, 53*(1), 28–35.

Department of Health. *Delivering high quality, effective, compassionate care: Developing the right people with the right skills and the right values.* 2013. https://assets.publishing.service.gov.uk/government/uploads/system/uploads/attachment_data/file/203332/29257_2900971_Delivering_Accessible.pdf

Edwards, N. (2005). *Birthing autonomy.* Routledge.

Feeley, C., & Thomson, G. (2016). Why do some women choose to freebirth in the UK? An interpretative phenomenological study. *BMC Pregnancy Childbirth, 16,* 59. https://doi.org/10.1186/s12884-016-0847-6.

Greenfield, M., Payne-Gifford, S., & McKenzie, G. (2021). Between a rock and a hard place: Considering "freebirth" during Covid-19. *Frontiers in Global Women's Health, 2,* 603744. https://doi.org/10.3389/fgwh.2021.603744.

Kirkham, M. (2010). The maternity services context. In Kirkham, M. (Ed.), *The midwife–mother relationship* (2nd ed., Chapter 1, pp. 3–11). Palgrave Macmillan.

MBRRACE-UK. *Mothers and babies: Reducing risk through audits and confidential enquiries across the UK.* 2021. https://www.npeu.ox.ac.uk/mbrrace-uk

McIntosh, T. (2012). *A social history of maternity care.* Routledge.

NHS England. *Better births. Improving outcomes of maternity services in England. A five year forward view for maternity care.* 2016. NHS England. https://www.england.nhs.uk/wp-content/uploads/2017/12/implementing-better-births.pdf

Ockenden D. *Independent review of maternity services at the Shrewsbury and Telford Hospital NHS Trust.* 2022. https://www.gov.uk/government/publications/final-report-of-the-ockenden-review

RCOG. *Birth after previous caesarean birth (Green-top guideline no. 45).* 2015. https://www.rcog.org.uk/en/guidelines-research-services/guidelines/gtg45/

Watson, J. (2009). Caring science and human caring theory: Transforming personal and professional practices of nursing and health care. *Journal of Health and Human Services Administration, 31*(4), 466–482.

## Resources

Birth Trauma Association: https://www.birthtraumaassociation.org.uk/
   *A charity which supports women who have experienced birth trauma. It primarily uses peer support.*

MBRRACE. *MBRRACE-UK: Mothers and babies: Reducing risk through audits and confidential enquiries across the UK.* https://www.npeu.ox.ac.uk/mbrrace-uk
   *The confidential enquiries into maternal death have existed in various forms since the 1930s. They are currently run by the NPEU (National Perinatal Epidemiology unit) which is a multidisciplinary research unit which was established at the University of Oxford in 1978.*

https://www.birthrights.org.uk/factsheets/unassisted-birth/
https://www.aims.org.uk/information/item/freebirth
   *Freebirth: Birthrights and AIMS both have information about freebirthing.*

# CHAPTER 9

# Communication Around Loss and Trauma

Rebekah Wells

## Introduction

When things go well in life it is not hard to congratulate someone and to celebrate with them. Pregnancy, birth and the postnatal period are perhaps the most celebrated phase of life for new and expanding families. Congratulations abound from the point of the pregnancy announcement and peak at the safe arrival of the newborn. Loss and trauma are the antithesis of birth and joy, pervasive powerful experiences that arguably require even more thoughtful communication and support than the comparably straightforward arrival of a newborn.

The role of the midwife encompasses a broad spectrum of clinical and practical skills necessary to support the physiological aspects of pregnancy, birth and the postnatal period. Alongside this the midwife also has a unique opportunity to support the wide-ranging experiences of the childbearing year in a compassionate and holistic manner, recognising the psychological and emotional components of pregnancy and birth. The key ingredient to the application of all of these skills in practice is communication, from the basics of introductions to the ways in which the details of complex situations are appropriately imparted, and through the nuances of how the room is lit or which tone of voice is adopted. These skills are always important and form the basis of quality midwifery practice, but when faced with supporting families[1] through unexpected experiences of loss or trauma the evidence is clear that what is said, and how it is said, can make a profound and lasting impact (Aldridge, 2008; Farrales et al., 2020).

This chapter will begin to explore communication around loss and trauma, starting by giving some thought to definitions and considering application to practice

---

[1] In the context of this chapter 'families' will be referred to frequently, more so than woman or birthing person, as the experiences of loss and trauma are widely acknowledged to affect more than the person who is pregnant or giving birth—there are no assumptions made or implied and it is intended that the word 'family' encompasses every iteration of family as defined by the family themselves.

throughout. The nature of both loss and trauma as unique and individually constructed experiences will be discussed[2], and the crucial role of individualised communication will be considered. Principles of confident, sensitive, respectful and clear communication will be elaborated on for application both in the midst of a loss or traumatic event and in the immediate aftermath. The role of counselling and debriefing in such situations will also be considered, and key skills for communicating with those who have had a previous experience of loss or trauma will be highlighted. Finally, the importance of communication for professionals in order to access their own support and debriefing will be explored.

---

**QUICK REFLECTION**

Consider an experience from practice that you would define as being traumatic in nature.
- What led you to defining the event as traumatic?
- Setting your own interpretation of the event as traumatic aside, would this have been seen as a traumatic event by
  - The person who was pregnant or giving birth?
  - Their partner or companion?
  - Your colleagues?

---

# Setting the Scene
## DEFINING LOSS AND TRAUMA

Defining loss and trauma is challenging—they are both intensely personal experiences and conceptualised in different ways from one person to the next. Exploring dictionary definitions would provide little or no insight into the experiences of individuals. Each person pregnant or giving birth, each companion in the birth or other clinical setting, and each midwife will construct their own meaning of loss and trauma.

Most commonly within midwifery loss is referring to perinatal baby loss or pregnancy loss. The broad spectrum of this in itself highlights the complexities in defining loss—from the earliest forms of loss such as an in vitro fertilisation (IVF) treatment cycle that doesn't develop into a pregnancy or an early miscarriage only days after a positive pregnancy test, right through to the death of a baby a few weeks old. There are stark contrasts in the physiological differences of these events

---

[2]This chapter will naturally touch on topics that could cause distress for some individuals. At the end of the chapter there are links for accessing support specific to those who have had any kind of pregnancy loss or baby loss, or those who have had a traumatic experience in pregnancy, childbirth or the postnatal period, whether or not they were the person pregnant or giving birth.

and in the social constructs of the tangible newborn bundle compared to the privacy of losing a pregnancy quietly and often alone. However, the magnitude of the grief experienced by the individual cannot be defined as simply as physiology (Diamond et al., 2021). Loss can also mean much more than loss of life and for many an experience of loss during the childbearing year will be a complex personal experience—a planned pregnancy that results in twins could create a sense of loss of normality; a planned elective Caesarean that is queue jumped by a precipitate spontaneous vaginal birth could lead to feeling a loss of control; a congenital abnormality diagnosed in pregnancy could induce a sense of loss of choice in birth preferences. Each individual will have a unique experience and every single personal construction of loss is valid and therefore considered interchangeably in this chapter.

Trauma can be more challenging to define than loss. Where loss has a literal meaning and then a complex personal interpretation and experience, trauma is subjective, meaning that identical pregnancy, birthing or postnatal experiences may be defined as traumatic by one person and not by another. The American Psychiatric Association (APA) acknowledge that trauma is individual, but they highlight key contributors to trauma as the influence of a disrupted sense of control, the impact of distress, and the experience of fear and helplessness (APA, 2013).

In the context of communication these very abstract definitions of loss and trauma begin to highlight the crucial nature of communication in the midwifery setting. Some instances of loss will be completely unavoidable but genuine and compassionate communication can contribute to the long-term psychological impact experienced. In terms of trauma, the role of the midwife offers a unique opportunity to minimise the impact of a traumatic experience—for example, supportive and tactful communication in the midst of things can mitigate the sense of fear and helplessness. Navigating instances of loss and trauma will be explored in more detail later in the chapter, and in addition skills for supporting those with a history of loss or trauma will be discussed.

## KEY PRINCIPLES

As other chapters will have already demonstrated, skilled and sensitive communication is integral to midwifery practice. When thinking specifically about communication around loss and trauma there are three key principles to keep front and centre of communication.

### The Value of Individualised Communication

Individualised care is central to high-quality midwifery practice, and this is true across every interaction throughout pregnancy, birth and the postnatal period. This is especially significant when thinking about loss and trauma, as we have already identified that these are intensely personal experiences in their construction and manifestation.

A mindful approach can aid individualised communication, as mindfulness incorporates notions of acceptance and nonjudgementalism and the suspension of personal assumptions (Cacciatore, 2017). Individual differences are a key feature of humanity, but in the context of midwifery communication, and especially in situations of trauma or loss, it is crucial to suspend personal norms and expectations when in the role of a caring professional. Approaching every conversation with families in an accepting and nonjudgemental way will not only establish the desire to communicate with them in an individualised way but ultimately will demonstrate a commitment to caring for them in a way that will best suit their individual needs.

All communication in the practice setting should be built upon principles of thoughtful individualised care, and such kindness should absolutely be universal. An example of the beneficial impact of truly individualised care and communication can be seen in the context of post-traumatic stress disorder (PTSD), which is a complex mental health condition that develops following traumatic events. As we have already seen, trauma is an individual experience, and not all traumatic events in the childbearing year will evolve into PTSD. There are of course many factors that will contribute to the individual response to trauma, but there is evidence that demonstrates the impact of preexisting vulnerabilities on the development of PTSD (Ayers et al., 2016). Applying knowledge of these existing vulnerabilities to enhance individualised care can contribute to reducing the long-term impacts of trauma and loss.

For every family experiencing loss or trauma there will not only be individual differences in processing the experience but also wider cultural influences. Cultural communication is explored more fully in another chapter within this book (Chapter 6), but it is important to highlight here in the context of loss and trauma. The personal construction of the experience of loss and trauma will for each individual include elements of their cultural identity, and this may not be the same cultural identity as experienced by those in the position of providing care. Taking care to individualise communication and care can ensure that the nuances of each individual family, including their cultural identity, are truly taken into account, and that their needs are met and respected as a priority over providing 'checklist' care (Farrales et al., 2020).

## Speaking Versus Silence

If you tell anyone that you are a midwife you will often quickly be met with the response 'oh how lovely, being part of such an exciting time for people'. There is obviously a great deal of truth in this and indeed not many midwives embark on their career with a particular interest in loss, trauma and the difficult conversations that surround those experiences. It can therefore be intensely difficult to know what to say when you are presented with those situations—the times when it is not exciting or joyful. Midwives practise history taking, labour support or congratulating after the safe arrival of a baby on a daily basis; responding in the event of loss and trauma is, thankfully in many ways, a less practised skill.

However, the research shows us that silence is one of the things that families find the hardest in instances of loss and trauma and this can lead to a feeling of isolation (Diamond et al., 2021). Blankly saying nothing at all can be a powerful form of communication in its own right and therefore saying something is an important part of demonstrating compassion. On occasions this can feel daunting and not knowing what to say can be the underlying issue rather than lack of compassion. A helpful first point on working out what to say is to engage in empathetic communication. Empathy is distinct from sympathy, and this is important in the context of loss and trauma. Empathetic communication is rooted in sharing understanding, seeing the situation through the other person's eyes. Sympathy, by contrast, is more about sharing emotions and often expressing sorrow or pity (Charitou et al., 2019). Empathetic understanding and communication can be key to self-expression in instances of trauma and loss. Coming alongside families in these moments is an important part of the role of a health care professional and showing emotion or expressing sadness demonstrates genuineness and compassion (Farrales et al., 2020). Acknowledging the sadness in a situation supports the family as they begin to navigate their own grief.

Of course there are times when silence can be ok, or even the best choice, and in these moments it is broader communication skills that come into their own—softening the environment by turning the lights down for a couple coming to terms with unexpected news, providing clean sheets and plumped pillows for the person who has just experienced a traumatic birth, proffering hot buttered toast for the mother trying to express milk for a baby in the neonatal intensive care unit (NICU).

Kindness, and its components such as attentiveness, compassion and thoughtfulness, can never be underrated and arguably forms valuable key characteristics for midwives (Moloney & Gair, 2015). Perhaps this can best be summarised as benevolence—that is, the quality of well-meaning. When faced with difficult situations and potentially awkward silences, bringing together benevolence and empathy will ensure that communication can not only be used to impart important details but to provide care and compassion for those finding themselves in an unexpected and distressing situation.

## Choosing Words

Having established that it is important to communicate one way or another with people in times of loss and trauma, it is no surprise to highlight that the content of what is said is important. Filling the silence with thoughtless words can contribute negatively to psychological wellbeing in the midst of loss or trauma, or when there has been a previous loss or trauma.

| Don't use platitudes such as... | Choose words carefully, swapping potentially insensitive ones for kinder options | Avoid throwaway remarks such as... |
|---|---|---|
| You've got through this you can get through anything. | Instead of 'failed' induction, try ineffective induction, or instead of 'failure to progress' try slowed labour. | At least you know you can get pregnant. |
| It could be worse. | If a stillborn baby has a name, use the name rather than simply referring to he/she/it. | No birth is perfect. |
| Time heals all wounds. | | There is always next time. |
| It wasn't meant to be. | | |
| Everything happens for a reason. | Avoid saying 'it's not your fault' as this can perpetuate a notion of blame. | Nature knows what it's doing. |

The application of empathy can come into its own when choosing what to say, or what not to say. Try thinking about how you might feel in a scenario of loss or trauma—what empathetic and understanding responses would you benefit from hearing in that situation? Or imagine the person is a close friend or relative of yours—what kind and compassionate words would you speak in this instance to a person for whom you cared deeply?

**PRACTICE POINTS**
- Be mindful that the individually constructed nature of loss and trauma may mean that an individual's experience doesn't look like loss or trauma 'on paper'.
- Carefully considering words and sentiments expressed is especially important in times of loss and trauma, but silence can be an isolating experience and communicating anything in an empathetic way is beneficial in such situations.

## In the Thick of It

**QUICK REFLECTION**
Think about a time when you encountered loss in the practice setting.
- How did the experience make you feel?
- Do you remember any of your communication to the family? If so
  - How do you think your communication contributed positively to their experience?
  - What would you change about how you communicated with them?

## DURING

As a midwife there is a great deal of communication that has to be conducted very swiftly in times of potential trauma or loss. There is the essential contemporaneous record keeping as stipulated by the Nursing and Midwifery Council (NMC, 2018) and there is the necessary transfer of knowledge from one staff member to another. There is also the crucial challenge of keeping those affected included in the discussion, up to date with events and reassured where appropriate. Importantly this is not restricted simply to the person who is pregnant or giving birth but includes their partner or birth companion, or wider family at times too. Record keeping and handover skills have been discussed in other chapters, as has information sharing with the person who is pregnant or giving birth. However, there are specific challenges associated with communicating with those in the midst of experiencing loss or trauma and we will consider those further here.

a. **Clarity is vital when information processing may be hard**—emotional responses are naturally high in instances of loss or trauma and therefore it is more important to carefully consider tone and terminology than in more run-of-the-mill exchanges. Health care professionals need to communicate in clear ways, consistent with the emotional state of the individual to increase the chance of them hearing and understanding what is being said (Druguet et al., 2019). This is especially important when decisions need to be made quickly, some of which will be irreversible.

b. **Don't make empty promises**—it is a human instinct to tell someone in distress that 'everything will be ok'. Within midwifery practice, though, these should be avoided at all costs as there is never any guarantee that things will be ok. In the event that things do not work out ok, these words can long ring in the ears of the family or of the midwife who said them. Instead, seek to offer support in concrete ways; for example, 'we will do everything we can to look after you and your baby' in a labour emergency is true.

c. **Describe things in an appropriate way for the individual**—it isn't always possible but wherever it is possible use your knowledge of the individual to tailor the way you explain things to them. This may include enhancing clarity by using terms easily understood by the general public, or conversely may include using medical language if that better meets the experience of the individual. Watch and listen to them as you are communicating in order to get a sense of whether they need more or less information or details and to gauge whether your tone and style is right for them.

d. **Involve the wider family as appropriate**—in times of loss and in potentially traumatic situations it can be helpful to include family when explaining things. In the midst of these unexpected and distressing experiences it can be challenging to hear information, and therefore including family in the conversations can aid the conveyance of important facts and increase decision-making capacity. Naturally this needs to be done sensitively and with consent.

e. **Saying 'don't worry' is futile and insensitive**—it is very tempting to say 'don't worry' to someone who is facing a difficult situation and on the surface this seems like a kind thing to say. However, not only is this insensitive as it diminishes the feelings being experienced by the individual, but it is completely futile as it actually goes against every human instinct. Humans are biologically wired to respond to stress, and worrying is part of a healthy human response to an unexpected or traumatic event. Instead focus on explaining the clinical, practical or emotional support that you and your colleagues are going to provide so that this will naturally reduce their sense of helplessness or distress.

f. **Be mindful of your professional communications in front of the family**—people listen when health care professionals talk to each other, and this includes family members as well as the person who is pregnant, giving birth or newly postnatal.

   ▪ Don't say anything that you would not be happy saying to the individual or family directly.
   ▪ Do not share new information between staff that has yet to have been discussed with the people affected.
   ▪ Avoid speaking in professional 'code' that excludes those being talked about.
   ▪ Remember that curtains are not walls.

## IN THE IMMEDIATE AFTERMATH

In the midst of loss or a traumatic experience, much of the communication taking place will be dictated by events, and although hopefully suffused with compassion, there will be many descriptive and functional exchanges. In the immediate aftermath there is an opportunity to communicate with those affected in ways that can ultimately reduce the long-term psychological distress. This can be achieved through sensitively and respectfully communicating with the family about the events that have just taken place, and this can be done in an empathetic way to ensure the information is shared as helpfully and kindly as possible. However, there is also a professional responsibility to be honest with people and to apologise when things go wrong (NMC, 2018). Saying sorry is an integral part of the professional Duty of Candour, but importantly this is not the same as accepting liability. It does, however, express regret for an outcome and acknowledges that things could have gone better (Care Quality Commission (CQC), 2021). For those who have experienced loss or trauma in the childbearing year a swift and genuine apology can be a significant contributor to reducing long-term psychological distress.

Communication is a two-way affair and a key component to communicating with people in the immediate aftermath of unexpected distressing events is to listen to them. For midwives, that could manifest as asking families what they understand of the events that have just taken place, enabling a more personalised immediate debrief. It could include simply asking them how they feel. For those who have experienced loss or trauma during pregnancy, birth or the postnatal period, when health care professionals adopt an open and nonjudgemental approach this can empower the individual or family to express more fully how they are feeling and what support they need. It would be easy to make decisions for people, or to decide what support they need, but the individual nature of loss and trauma experiences highlights the necessity to not only include those affected in the conversation but to actually put them at the centre.

Specifically in the context of loss, which we have already defined as an intensely personal experience, it is important to acknowledge that grief is a healthy response. Supporting this is a key responsibility of health professionals to enable people to process the experience (Burden et al., 2016) and this can, and should, begin immediately. The specifics of the loss experience are essentially irrelevant, and to provide holistic, individualised care it is essential to take the lead from the person themselves. Loss, and the grief associated with it, can often get missed in the midst of physiological definitions and administrative details (Diamond et al., 2021) and therefore being sensitive to the individual's interpretation of events and communicating in a way that is in keeping with their experience will ensure compassionate communication.

In considering communication in the immediate aftermath of trauma, it is useful to think back to the definition of trauma—that is, there is no definition of trauma because it is a subjective experience, constructed by the individual experiencing it. A traumatic birth, for example, arises from the subjective perception of events in the course of the birth process (Andersen et al., 2012) which contains no specifics about what has to occur, or not occur, in order to define it as traumatic. This can be confronting for midwives to understand as each will naturally have their own construct of what constitutes a traumatic birth experience. However, assimilating the concept of trauma as subjective into midwifery practice can actually improve communication when supporting those who have experienced trauma. The role of the midwife is not to tell the person who has just given birth that it wasn't traumatic, but to acknowledge their trauma as subjective, support them in their experience and never to take it personally.

## SENSITIVE PRACTICE FOLLOWING PREVIOUS LOSS OR TRAUMA

Sensitive and individualised practice is synonymous with good midwifery care, but there will always be instances in practice that require explicitly sensitive care. For those who have experienced loss or trauma in a previous pregnancy, birth or the postnatal period, facing the experiences again with a subsequent pregnancy will likely cause a complex mix of emotions. Midwives are uniquely placed to offer support in this situation and the content and tone of their communication undoubtedly have an impact on this new, and potentially positive, experience. Key principles for communication in a subsequent pregnancy can be considered separately for trauma, loss and additionally for previous nonperinatal loss.

## Trauma

As already highlighted, trauma is subjective. When meeting someone in a subsequent pregnancy they are entitled to define their previous experience as traumatic whether you think it looks traumatic 'on paper' or not.

### PRACTICE POINTS

- Does your clinical practice area have a way of obviously highlighting previous trauma on medical notes?
- Evidence shows us that continually having to re-tell the trauma to every medical professional can compound the trauma (Diamond et al., 2021).

Being mindful in your communication with someone with a history of birth or pregnancy trauma will ensure that you take on board their interpretation and support their experience. The principle of empathy can be helpful in this instance by working to see the situation through the other person's eyes—as a midwife, suspending your own belief about what constitutes trauma is crucial in accepting the individual's experience. This in turn will ensure positive and individualised care for a subsequent pregnancy.

Many people who have experienced trauma in a previous pregnancy or birth will have a clear idea about what they feel was traumatic and therefore what they want and need in terms of both process and communication this time round. Others will have a less clear idea about the specifics of the traumatic experience. In either case it is important to understand the experience from the perspective of those affected, and to together explore the options for future care. Asking sensitive questions, listening attentively and accepting the perceptions of the family are key to providing compassionate support following trauma (Gamble & Creedy, 2009).

## Loss

Although loss is a complex and personally constructed experience, a key feature of any loss experience is grief. Acknowledging this is important in subsequent pregnancies for those who have previously experienced loss and demonstrates empathetic understanding. For those who have experienced the loss of a baby in pregnancy, accepting their grief and understanding the fact that that baby was irreplaceable is paramount (Farrales et al., 2020). Pregnancy and baby loss can cause parents to feel isolated and outside the boundaries of normality (Burden et al., 2016), which can be particularly acute during a subsequent pregnancy. Taking care to include pregnancies that have concluded in loss when talking about parity or birth order, for example, demonstrates that their previous experience is valid and important.

Although loss is unquestionably stressful and traumatic, everyone who encounters it will experience it differently (Druguet et al., 2019), which further highlights the importance of individualised communication. Previous pregnancy loss is known as a risk factor for antenatal anxiety (Bayrampour et al., 2018), which is essential to keep in mind when caring for families who are in a subsequent pregnancy—fears may be elevated, and communication needs to be tailored to respond in a helpful and empathetic way.

## Subsequent Pregnancies and Births After the Loss of a Baby or Child

This chapter has focused on communication around loss during pregnancy or childbirth and baby loss, but in caring for families in subsequent pregnancies it is important to be mindful of those who don't fit that category. Families who have experienced the death of a child outside of the perinatal period will have an equally complex mix of emotions but often miss out on support and can feel that they have experienced 'the wrong kind of loss'. The following highlights some helpful guidance when supporting families in this unique situation.

| | |
|---|---|
| Be mindful that the death of a child permeates the whole of life. | For a parent to lose a child is against the natural order and can therefore disrupt all assumptions held about life. |
| Avoid generalised reassurances—acknowledge risks and offer support. | Families who have experienced the death of a baby or child are deprived of that innocence in simply trusting that all will be ok. |
| Do not brush off seemingly mild concerns. | Elements of everyday midwifery practice such as physiological jaundice or newborn weight loss may be magnified as concerns for those who have previously had a child who died. |
| Never imply that a new baby makes up for a child who has died. | Acknowledging the child who has died will allow the family to explore the juxtaposition of grief and joy. |
| Understand that parents will always be parenting their deceased child. | Supporting parents through a subsequent pregnancy or birth includes empowering them to parent both the child in their heart and the baby in their arms. |
| Ask inclusive questions. | Remember always to include them when talking about parity, family size and birth order. |
| Embrace and indulge conversations about the child that has died. | Ask them about the child, **always** ask their name. Take your lead from the family and be sensitive, but most families express this as a wonderful way of keeping the child part of everyday life. |

| Be mindful of families feeling they have experienced the 'wrong kind of loss'. | The maternity services are more familiar with perinatal or pregnancy loss and this can be alienating for families. |
| Don't consider prolonged grief unusual or pathological. | It is important to acknowledge and accept the long-term grief families experience as a product of their endless love. Supporting this will enhance their future experiences of pregnancy or birth. |

Modified from Wells (2020).

### PRACTICE POINTS

- Take the time and care to communicate in a way that meets the emotional needs of the individual or family because this can have a positive effect on the psychological impact of the event.
- Saying sorry is always the right thing to do when things go wrong. It does not imply any liability but humanly acknowledges a poor outcome.
- The experience of loss or trauma is personally constructed. Remember this for subsequent pregnancies and respect the interpretation of the story as told by the family.

# Debriefing and Counselling

Loss and trauma by very definition are adverse experiences in life, unexpected in nature and often causing a degree of psychological distress. In the context of antenatal, birth and postnatal care this is an important point to acknowledge—psychological distress as a response to loss or trauma should be considered a normal response. This means that timely support should be provided without the need for mental health assessment (Ockenden, 2022). In the immediate aftermath, as already highlighted, midwives are uniquely placed to offer the earliest forms of debriefing and counselling, but knowledge of specialist support services and prompt referral to these are important after loss and trauma.

### QUICK REFLECTION

Following loss or trauma in pregnancy, childbirth or the postnatal period, consider the role of debriefing and counselling.
- When do you think these should happen?
- Who do you think should facilitate them?
- What do you know about available options in your practice area?

Counselling can be an integral component of the grieving process in instances of both loss and trauma. Counselling has been covered in depth in its own chapter within this book, but there are aspects of counselling that are useful to consider for all health professionals when communicating with families following loss or trauma. Five key themes that can contribute to helpful counselling following perinatal loss include 'compassion and understanding; nonjudgemental; accepting of emotional state; deep listening and a place of narration; processing of emotion and perspective' (Cacciatore, 2017, p. 644). Essentially this highlights the importance of the mindful and empathetic communication considered earlier. It also emphasises the need to approach conversations in a truly individualised way, empowering families to tell their story without any judgement. A central feature in debriefing and counselling after trauma rests with acceptance of the perceptions of the individual (Gamble & Creedy, 2009). For midwives that can be an uncomfortable position to be in as the professional perspective of events may be markedly different. However, putting that interpretation aside and actively accepting the interpretation of events expressed by the individual or family as their truth is an important part of the process and will ultimately contribute to their recovery from the trauma.

In the event of stillbirth or pregnancy loss, whatever the gestation, making memory boxes and creating keepsakes can be an important part of the grieving process. When a baby dies before it is born it is immensely important to create these memories as there are no existing memories for families to carry with them (Aldridge, 2008). Every family will have a unique journey through perinatal loss, and it is important to respect that. This will be unexpected and uncharted territory for the family and therefore they will be looking for knowledgeable guidance and support as they make difficult decisions and begin to navigate their grief. Although compassionate support in the immediate aftermath is essential, long-term support services also play an important role in the grief process after perinatal bereavement. While prolonged grief should not be considered unusual or pathological, the impact of continued grief can be minimised by ongoing compassionate bereavement support services (Inati et al., 2018).

**PRACTICE POINTS**

- Applying nonjudgemental counselling skills to early communication following trauma or loss will support families as they begin to navigate their grief.
- Proactively supporting families to access the best form of debriefing or counselling for them is a key role for midwives following loss or trauma in pregnancy, birth or the postnatal period.

# Professional Support, Debriefing and Resilience

**QUICK REFLECTION**

Think of a time when you have encountered loss in the practice setting.
• How did the experience make you feel?
• Were you offered any debriefing or support?
• Did you take any time to informally reflect on the event?
• Would you know who to approach for support in the future?

It would not be appropriate to talk about communication around loss and trauma without including considerations of these experiences from a professional perspective. Communication for professionals is an integral part of psychological wellbeing, especially in the case of navigating the sometimes heartbreaking experiences of loss and trauma in a pregnancy and birth context. Contrary to an often-implied image, midwives are not superhuman—the capacity to seek help and support is not only an important professional characteristic but also an essential and extremely healthy one (Pezaro et al., 2016). Furthermore, the building and maintenance of professional confidence require effective support for midwives in practice—support is not a luxury, it is a necessity (Bedwell et al., 2015).

Professional support or supervision of one form or another has existed within the midwifery profession since 1902. The most recent approach promotes the role of the professional midwifery advocate (PMA) and the application of the A-Equip (Advocating for Education and Quality Improvement) model (NHS England, 2017), though this is neither statutory nor universally adopted. One of the four functions of the A-Equip model is 'restorative', which is aimed at providing support to improve wellbeing. Provision of support will vary from one setting to the next, but communicating a personal need for support, whether is it professional, emotional or spiritual, is an integral part of practice and for ensuring personal and professional wellbeing.

Across health professions, the concept of resilience is often referred to with regards to professional wellbeing, mental health and staff morale in a practice setting. The core notion of resilience is the capacity of a (thing or) person to experience some form of distress and to bounce back (Crowther et al., 2016). Within midwifery this is perhaps particularly pertinent in the instances of loss and trauma, as these are the aspects of practice that can elicit the greatest instances of distress for midwives. Providing professional care and support for those pregnant and giving birth can be challenging and hard work, but it is the unexpected poor outcomes that bring with them distress and require midwives to have resilience.

**PRACTICE POINTS**

- It is a professional strength to seek out support and to reflect on difficult experiences in practice, and this will actually improve confidence.
- Familiarise yourself with the support systems in place in your practice setting so that you know how to access support when the need arises.

# Conclusion

Key points from the chapter:

1. Trauma is subjective. Never decide for someone whether their experience is traumatic or not. Listen empathetically to their individual experience and respond with acceptance and kindness.
2. Loss can be about more than the loss of a pregnancy or the death of a baby, but will always result in grief. Acknowledging the essential role of grief and mindfully communicating with families will ensure that their unique experiences are respected and that their individual needs are met.
3. Individualised, respectful and honest communication is important for everyone involved—the person who is pregnant, postnatal or giving birth, the partner or companion, and the wider family. Loss and trauma are unexpected and distressing experiences, but sensitive communication can reduce the long-term psychological impact.

This chapter has begun to explore communication around loss and trauma. It has highlighted that both are complex and individual in their construction and definition and communication needs to reflect that. Principles of empathetic understanding and mindful communication have been explored as key skills for midwives and health care professionals when supporting families in times of loss and trauma. Above all this chapter has emphasised that kindness and compassion are essential skills for midwives when supporting families through times of distress. Though midwives may have no influence over the processes or outcomes, the quality of their communication is an integral cog in mitigating the psychological distress felt by families following loss or trauma.

## References

Aldridge, A. (2008). Perinatal loss—A life-changing experience. *Bereavement Care, 27*(2), 23–26.

Andersen, L. B., Melvaer, L. B., Videbech, P., Lamont, R. F., & Joergensen, J. S. (2012). Risk factors for developing post-traumatic stress disorder following childbirth: A systematic review. *Nordic Federation of Societies of Obstetrics and Gynecology, 91*(11), 1261–1272.

APA. (2013). *Diagnostic and statistical manual of mental disorders* (5th ed.). American Psychiatric Association.

Ayers, S., Bond, R., Bertullies, S., & Wijma, K. (2016). The aetiology of post-traumatic stress following childbirth: A meta-analysis and theoretical framework. *Psychological Medicine*, *46*(6), 1121–1134.

Bayrampour, H., Vinturache, A., Hetherington, E., Lorenzetti, D. L., & Tough, S. (2018). Risk factors for antenatal anxiety: A systematic review of the literature. *Journal of Reproductive and Infant Psychology*, *36*(5), 476–503.

Bedwell, C., McGowan, L., & Lavender, D. T. (2015). Factors affecting midwives' confidence in intrapartum care: A phenomenological study. *Midwifery*, *31*(1), 170–176.

Burden, C., Bradley, S., Storey, C., Ellis, A., Heazell, A. E. P., Downe, S., Cacciatore, J., & Siassakos, D. (2016). From grief, guilt pain and stigma to hope and pride – A systematic review and meta-analysis of mixed-method research of the psychosocial impact of still-birth. *BMC Pregnancy Childbirth*, *16*, 9. https://doi.org/10.1186/s12884-016-0800-8.

Cacciatore, J. (2017). 'She used his name': Provider trait mindfulness in perinatal death counselling. *Studies in Psychology*, *38*(3), 639–666.

Charitou, A., Fifli, P., & Vivilaki, V. G. (2019). Is empathy an important attribute of mid-wives and other health professionals? A review. *European Journal of Midwifery*, *3*, 4. https://doi.org/10.18332/ejm/100612.

CQC. (2021). *The duty of candour: guidance for providers*. Care Quality Commission. https://www.cqc.org.uk/sites/default/files/20210421%20The%20duty%20of%20candour%20-%20guidance%20for%20providers.pdf. Accessed 12 April 2022.

Crowther, S., Hunter, B., McAra-Couper, J., Warren, L., Gilkison, A., Hunter, M., Fielder, A., & Kirkham, M. (2016). Sustainability and resilience in midwifery: A discussion paper. *Midwifery*, *40*, 40–48.

Diamond, R., Chou, J. L., & Bonis, S. (2021). Invisible loss: A Delphi approach to develop a term for individuals who experienced perinatal loss. *Journal of Feminist Family Therapy*, *33*(1), 81–100.

Druguet, M., Nuño, L., Rodó, C., Arévalo, S., Carreras, E., & Gómez-Benito, J. (2019). Influence of farewell rituals and psychological vulnerability on grief following perinatal loss in monochorionic twin pregnancy. *The Journal of Maternal-Fetal & Neonatal Medicine*, *32*(6), 1033–1035.

Farrales, L. L., Cacciatore, J., Jonas-Simpson, C., Dharamsi, S., Ascher, J., & Klein, M. C. (2020). What bereaved parents want health care providers to know when their babies are stillborn: A community-based participatory study. *BMC Psychology*, *8*, 18. https://doi.org/10.1186/s40359-020-0385-x.

Gamble, J., & Creedy, D. K. (2009). A counselling model for postpartum women after dis-tressing birth experiences. *Midwifery*, *25*(2), 21–30.

Inati, V., Matic, M., Phillips, C., Maconachie, N., Vanderhook, F., & Kent, A. L. (2018). A survey of the experiences of families with bereavement support services following a peri-natal loss. *The Australian & New Zealand Journal of Obstetrics & Gynaecology*, *58*(1), 54–63.

Moloney, S., & Gair, S. (2015). Empathy and spiritual care in midwifery practice: Contributing to women's enhanced birth experiences. *Women and Birth: Journal of the Australian College of Midwives*, *28*(4), 323–328.

NHS England. (2017). *A-EQUIP a model of clinical midwifery supervision*. NHS England. https://www.england.nhs.uk/wp-content/uploads/2017/04/a-equip-midwifery-supervi-sion-model.pdf. Accessed 12 April 2022.

NMC. (2018). *The Code: Professional standards of practice and behaviour for nurses, midwives and nursing associates*. NMC. https://www.nmc.org.uk/globalassets/sitedocuments/nmc-publications/nmc-code.pdf. Accessed 12 April 2022.

Ockenden, D. (2022). *Ockenden report – Final: Findings, conclusions and essential actions from the independent review of maternity services at The Shrewsbury and Telford Hospital NHS Trust*. Her Majesty's Stationery Office (HMSO). https://assets.publishing.service.gov.uk/government/uploads/system/uploads/attachment_data/file/1064302/Final-Ockenden-Report-web-accessible.pdf. Accessed 12 April 2022.

Pezaro, S., Clyne, W., Turner, A., Fulton, E. A., & Gerada, C. (2016). 'Midwives overboard!' Inside their hearts are breaking, their makeup may be flaking but their smile still stays on. *Women and Birth*, *29*(3), 59–66.

Wells, R. (2020). Child bereavement and subsequent parenting: Some key ideas for postnatal support. *The Practising Midwife*, *23*(2), 32–34.

## Resources

*There are numerous charities and organisations dedicated to supporting those who have experienced loss or trauma in the childbearing year; some also offer support for professionals. The following is a nonexhaustive selection; any recommendations to families would need to take individual situations and needs into account.*

**Antenatal Results and Choices (ARC)** offers information and support to parents in relation to antenatal screening, anomaly diagnoses, difficult decisions in pregnancy and bereavement.

Helpline: 0845 077 2290 or 0207 713 7486 (Monday–Friday, from 10:00 a.m. until 5:30 p.m.)

Email: info@arc-uk.org

Website: www.arc-uk.org

**Birth Trauma Association** is a charity focused on supporting those who specifically develop PTSD following a traumatic birth experience.

Email: support@birthtraumaassociation.org.uk

Website: https://www.birthtraumaassociation.org.uk/

**Miscarriage Association** offers support and information for anyone affected by the loss of a baby in early pregnancy.

Helpline: 01924 200799 (Monday–Friday, from 9:00 a.m. to 4:00 p.m.)

Email: info@miscarriageassociation.org.uk

Website: https://www.miscarriageassociation.org.uk/

**PANDAS Foundation** is a charity that supports those experiencing perinatal mental illness including pre- and postnatal anxiety and depression.

Helpline: 0808 1961 776

Website: https://pandasfoundation.org.uk/

**Peanut** is an organisation aimed at connecting women with other women at similar life stages. They recently championed the rewording of some language used in maternity and obstetric settings in the Renaming Revolution Glossary, which contains a selection of regularly used terms alongside more thoughtful alternatives.

https://www.peanut-app.io/blog/renaming-revolution-glossary

**Petals** is a baby loss counselling charity providing free-of-charge specialist counselling for anyone who experiences pregnancy or baby loss.

Email: counselling@petalscharity.org

Website: www.petalscharity.org

**Samaritans** are a registered charity for supporting anyone in distress 24 hours a day, 7 days a week.

Telephone: 116 123

Email: jo@samaritans.org

Website: www.samaritans.org

**SANDS** is the leading stillbirth and neonatal death charity in the UK. They aim to ensure that anyone experiencing the death of a baby receives the best possible care and support.

Website: https://www.sands.org.uk/

SANDS also has information on sensitive communication for professionals.

https://sands.org.uk/sites/default/files/Sensitive%20and%20Effective%20Communication.pdf

PART 3

# Communication in Practice

# CHAPTER 10

# Pregnancy

Ray Wild

## #Hellomynameis

Hello, my name is Rachel, but you can call me Ray.

I'm your guide for this chapter, which is about communication and the pregnancy journey. I'd like to start by telling you a little about myself, and what to expect for the next few pages. I'm a registered midwife and a midwifery educator, and I currently work as a health care lecturer. I have structured this chapter as a dialogue between colleagues, with the assumption you are also a midwife, learning to be one or working in the maternity services in some capacity.

First, I explore some key ideas about human communication and how it relates to everyday antenatal midwifery care. Many ideas I discuss apply throughout perinatal care; I focus on specific events in antenatal care where I think they are most obvious and familiar—the booking, screening and birth plans. I discuss and offer tips about communication between midwives and childbearing women and people; co-parents and wider support networks; and our colleagues in perinatal services and beyond. I also ask a lot of questions. Because I am communicating with you in writing I cannot personalise the information I am presenting, but I want you to know that I think of you as somebody with ideas and answers of your own. What you do with this chapter is ultimately for you to decide.

## Departures

Hello again, thanks for reading on. I have mapped out this chapter using an image we are all familiar with—pregnancy as a journey. Alongside the pregnant woman or person's journey, I hope to explore our journeys as midwives, and how there can be a mismatch between the two perspectives.

Think of this next section as packing a midwifery communication kitbag with me before we set off. As we travel, I present opportunities to reflect on midwifery practice and ourselves. If that gets uncomfortable at times, then I encourage slow thinking, taking a break and returning to the material at a pace that is challenging but manageable. Opportunities to slow down in midwifery can be rare and that

155

means they are precious. At times I will wander off into unfamiliar rough ground at the side of the road. My guess is you have an adventurous and curious mind, or you wouldn't have chosen to read this book. I hope you enjoy the adventure.

Now, so I can explain some of my key ideas about communication, I am going to share with you some information about myself that you might not notice from reading what I write. I am autistic, and that means my thinking and my communication are 'atypical'. Now, this isn't a chapter about me or about neurodiversity; it's a chapter about us, about midwives—but thinking about what elements of human cognition and communication are typical and atypical can be a useful method for us to explore communication in midwifery practice together.

- **Key idea 1: How we communicate feels like who we are. Changing how we communicate can disrupt our sense of self.**

For most people, interpersonal communication is like breathing. It's not something we think about unless we are making a special effort to bring it under conscious control, such as to meditate or swim under water. We find communicating straightforward unless it becomes strained; for example, because an interaction is not going well and we feel threatened, or disrespected, or misunderstood.

Language acquisition, including how we interpret body language and social meanings, happens in the very earliest months and years of our lives. The process is instinctive and developmental. After infancy the interactive aspects of communication, the back and forth of sharing meanings, are largely happening at a subconscious level, especially in familiar situations. Have a look at Chapter 3 on Principles of Communication to explore some of these ideas in more detail.

We do learn by about 18 months that what we are communicating affects others and we gain skills in how to moderate some of what we present. We soon learn how to choose to lie, to flatter, to comfort or to persuade. Even so we are processing complex messages and negotiations, impressions about levels of pleasantness or threat, without an awareness we are doing so.

Because I am autistic, I experience communication barriers and dissonance (a lack of harmony) in my communications with 'neurotypical' people more often than with other autistic people. I think a lot about the mechanics of how communication is done, because most of the time I am with people who are communicating differently to me. I describe what I do in these situations as communication on the manual setting, not on autopilot. As well as my communication itself, I'm often consciously thinking about what I am doing.

As midwives, we need to communicate across differences of which neurodivergence is only one type. If we do not share a language, culture or class background with someone we are providing care for, we may need to consciously alter what we communicate and how. The evidence that we often do this poorly is clear. Black women and people report consistently not being listened to or respected by White midwives. This is a major avoidable harm that has significantly contributed to the four to five times higher rates of death during childbearing for Black women (MBRRACE, 2021). If you are a person of colour this is not going to be new information, and I'm sorry for the ongoing stress and worry that racism in health care will have caused you. If like me you are White, then I'd like to invite you to think about some of the communication about inequality we are used to hearing. I was involved in national NHS meetings shortly after the 2019 MBRRACE (MBRRACE, 2021) Confidential Enquiry into Maternal Death identified the persistent inequity in maternal deaths for Black women. At this time implicit bias in health care had led to a dominant pattern of communication where clinicians were looking for physiological or social circumstances that had caused more deaths. It was only through the persistent advocacy of Black women, and other people of colour, that racism is now identified as the cause of harm. Chapter 6 talks in more detail about communicating sensitively in circumstances we may not be familiar with.

In perinatal care interactions, midwives are usually on home ground. Keeping our thinking on manual and processing our emotions appropriately can be draining, especially in services that are based on heavy workloads, clinics with set schedules and long shifts. During antenatal care midwives are communicating what pregnant women and people can expect from care during birth and afterwards. We can encourage autonomy, self-efficacy and trust—or we can teach people to expect little, and plan for self-preservation.

- **Key idea 2: When we become aware of miscommunication, humans are prone to blame the other person, but midwives are responsible for improving communication by reflecting on our personal feelings.**

When humans become aware of miscommunication it feels unpleasant. We can unconsciously experience communication barriers as aspects of the other person's self, rather than a puzzle to be solved by two equals.

## COFFEE BREAK ACTIVITY

Take a highlighter and go through the previous section. What parts, if any, remind you of midwifery communication?
- Greetings
- Framing
- Planning
- Personalisation
- Choice
- Information giving
- Explaining
- Consent
- Disclosure
- Challenge

Putting communication on the manual setting can be an advantage in these situations; however, for many people it will be a skill only developed as part of becoming a health care professional. Consciously reflecting on communication may feel laborious and end up reserved for formal communication such as SBAR (situation, background, assessment, recommendations), shift handovers or emergency protocols and safety checklists.

I'm going to ask you to slow down and reflect as we go along, because slow thinking, with time to process what we feel, can help us to be open to learning and change and increase empathy.

## Beginnings: Bookings

I'm sure many of you will have memories of your own experiences of maternity care. I'd like you to put that aside for a short while and think instead about your first day learning to be a midwife in clinical practice. Midwifery training and mentorship have changed over time, but it is essentially a 1:1 process of enculturation as well as clinical education, and this holds true across many health care systems internationally. On my first day at a small hospital in England, I was scheduled to meet my mentor for a placement on an antenatal ward, but she had been transferred to the operating theatre. About an hour later I was in scrubs, in a sluice, being taught how to identify the completeness of a placenta. I have no memory whatsoever of the person who had just given birth, or the person who had just been born.

The beginnings that most of us as student midwives have (or are having now) are about learning how to fit in with our mentors and a wider team of staff. We learn by 'see one, do one', and we learn to do it quickly. We learn how to speak as they do, present ourselves as they do, even if we aspire to do things differently. Childbearing women and people are visitors in our world. Even when we do the actual visiting, we control the encounters—the timing and content of visits, the flow of information and education. In many care models we will decide the timing and structure of interactions, even in a person's own home. We begin our midwifery journey in a setting where our survival depends more on our relationship with a midwifery team than on our relationships with people we are caring for. In many cases this will continue throughout our careers.

It is at this point that we reach a crossroads in our discussion.

I hope you are feeling a little confused. Possibly you are scribbling in the margins of your book or crossly typing into your e-reader something like 'Ah, but what about Continuity?'

Let me take you on a little detour. Between 2016 and 2021 I worked nationally and locally to design and set up continuity models of midwifery care. I also taught services about implementing continuity, and supported online about 2000 service users, midwives and doctors. Continuity midwifery does many things to positively change the power dynamics and communication between midwives and the women and people we work for. But continuity is not a magic wand to change the culture and orientation of services until it becomes, as the NHS in England intends, the default model of care. Even when that happens, most midwives will still have been trained and worked in 'discontinuity-based' service-oriented environments. We can take midwives out of fractured care, but can we take fractured care out of midwives? We can see how conditional models of continuity are by the way that the Ockenden Report (Ockenden, 2022) has side-lined them. Continuity has become an aspiration to be developed once other problems in maternity care have been solved rather than being seen as a fundamental element of personal, safe responsive care.

## Case Study

You now have two paths in front of you.

- To the left you are going to do a prebooking visit with Farhana who has accepted the standard Group Midwife Practice pathway. You have been invited to her home at 17:00 when her husband Riz will be up before his night shift. Farhana was helpful in getting her favourite BSL (British Sign Language) interpreter to come at that time, which is perfect because your signing is pretty basic. Everyone gets at least one prebooking visit, and this way you can all check the three-way communication will be good enough to take a full obstetric and social history. Tomorrow you will let the team know on WhatsApp if this family has accepted you for their booking, or if you need to jiggle things round to offer an alternative caseload.
- To the right you are going to a booking clinic at a GP surgery. You have three booking packs, two of which are for colleagues' caseloads. Letters have been sent for 9:30 (that one is yours), 10:30 and 11:45 because the second one is booking late after not attending previous appointments. The GP referral says they only speak Tigrigna, Italian and Arabic, so you hope an interpreter shows up. If you set off now you will be able to check whether the booking bloods are back from the maternity support worker's drop-in clinic, which saves a lot of time.
- Take 15–20 minutes. Have a snack. Make private notes about how you would approach these two different bookings to maximise positive communication and build trust in that setting.
- Turn the paper over. Now make notes about what you would really do.

NICE guidance (NICE, 2021) currently lists 50 separate topics for discussion and shared decision-making in the first booking appointment. Fifteen are topics I would characterise as sensitive, complex, potentially distressing or stigmatising. These include broad topics such as mental health issues, domestic abuse, obstetric and medical history, weight, smoking, drug use and alcohol intake, and risk of female genital mutilation (FGM). Each of these requires tact, sensitivity and a high level of skill in listening and understanding. This can include an awareness not just of what is being said, but also what is not being said. What are the gaps? Are there areas that the client seems unwilling to discuss? Even more importantly, if they raise issues or concerns, do you have the time and space to acknowledge them and to listen properly before speaking?

The documentation we use for booking and our anxiety not to forget anything can reduce the encounter to a stilted formulaic question-and-answer session. The trick is to be personal and to listen actively while also capturing the information required to understand the broad clinical picture. This means being flexible in how we carry out our booking conversations. It is tempting to attempt to have all the information at once— both in terms of firing questions at the family and in terms of transmitting information about place of birth, infant feeding, healthy eating or smoking cessation. Both parties can leave the appointment feeling confused and overwhelmed. It can be valuable to break the information and to really think about what key information and idea and conversation need to happen at booking and which ones can wait until further on into the pregnancy and the midwife–parent relationship. It may be that a woman does not feel comfortable disclosing sensitive details at booking when she has never met you before, but by 28 weeks feels ready to trust you with details of FGM or domestic abuse.

Clearly both foregoing scenarios presented will give pregnant people and families the information they need at the beginning of their pregnancy and will begin to lay the foundations of clinical care. In Farhana's case it seems clear the relationship has begun on a personal respectful and enabling level. By choosing her own interpreter and the timing of the meeting, Farhana already has some control over how the communication and therefore what the relationship between her and the maternity service will look like. In the second scenario it appears that care and communication are task driven and organised around the service rather than around families. Nevertheless, even in this situation care and communication can be humanised and personalised. This can be achieved in really simple ways by thinking about how we greet people, what we say, and what we show in our stance and body language before midwifery care or conversations even commence.

## THE COMMUNITY OF FAMILY

### QUICK REFLECTION

Notice your first response and then notice your second thoughts:
- Is midwifery a service for fathers?
- Is a newborn baby your patient?
- Do you speak to babies before they are born?
- If midwifery is woman centred what does that mean for women who are the baby's other mother?
- Is a man who is pregnant a father?
- Is a pregnant woman's male partner expecting a baby?
- What if the baby's biological father is someone else?
- Do you feel differently if this is because of donor insemination or a sexual relationship?

When I lecture or give talks about maternity services, I often ask people in the audience to raise a hand if they have ever been a baby. While this is useful to make people laugh, I am also entirely serious. Most of us first use maternity services when we are born rather than when we are giving birth. In English we say parents are 'expecting'. We might send a card wishing a newborn baby a 'welcome to the world'. I want you to take a moment to think about who you are a midwife to, and who midwifery is for.

Humans are a social species, and so from birth we are developing a sensitivity to the communication of welcome and belonging. This is connected to our basic survival needs because human infants cannot survive alone, and few adults thrive in isolation. As midwives in Britain, we acknowledge that a baby is not legally a person until they are born and that our first responsibility is to the person who is pregnant. This is vital to protect each childbearing person's bodily autonomy and is not true in every country. Throughout this chapter I have usually referred to people who are pregnant as 'childbearing people' for two reasons. In this context I am aiming to communicate that when women are pregnant, they are individual people, and I am hoping to use gender-neutral language to affirm that pregnant people are not always women.

Purposeful use of unfamiliar language can help with our thinking, but it can be alienating and confusing in practice. We need to pay attention to how communication of welcome and belonging is experienced, not how we want it to be understood. Within the context of maternity care, most fathers will not understand the word 'parent' to mean father, and most people will not understand the word 'partner' to mean they are being addressed as a father, mother or co-parent.

As time goes on and people move through their pregnancy they maybe begin to understand and to decode the language we use. This includes not just the clinical language of palpations and observation, but our forms of address and organisation. A father may gradually realise that the word 'partner' refers to him just as the pregnant person may begin to see how the work of sonographers, support workers, midwives and obstetricians dovetails to make a complete service.

Finally, in relation to our booking case studies we need to remember that because everyone is different, we cannot assume that the type of interaction we might like or value for ourselves will be right for other people. Some people will want and need continuity of care models and a really personal touch. Others might prefer the relationship to be more 'professional' and scientific in approach. However care is organised, take your communication cues from families you are meeting. Remember to keep your communication senses switched to 'manual' and observe and listen. Across three booking appointments you may find that your language and tone vary. This is not to say that some people are getting a better service than others but that your communication is thoughtful and responsive rather than taking a 'one size fits all' approach.

## THE ENVIRONMENT OF CARE

I sometimes used to sit in a small café next to a birth centre where I used to work and think about the meaning of welcome. Inside the birth centre I knew much care and attention had gone into how people were greeted in both the physical design and the staff's actions.

I was usually there to meet a midwifery colleague to talk about the service improvement projects I was involved in. At this time, I had moved from clinical practice into a multiprofessional team of people who were investigating, designing and testing what support might help families from the early weeks of pregnancy until the children went to school.

If I zoom out in my mind right now, I can clearly see the layout of the whole building and it has become a personal metaphor for me about how maternity services communicate who they are for, who is welcome and when. Of course, different hospitals in Britain, different hospitals across the world, do not have a single way to arrange their clinical estate, but we communicate welcome and a right to be somewhere by words, by décor, by the layout of a building, by even the signs and the doors and the arrangement of furniture.

From where I sit in the café, I often see fathers arriving to visit the wards upstairs or carrying their baby in a car seat for their first trip home. Some are clutching letters trying to find the scan department. Sometimes I see a man with his labouring partner arriving at the birth centre or the labour ward down the corridor. Some of the staff are male, including a small minority of the midwives and support workers, but everywhere there are women who are not here for the maternity services. The women who need a termination of their pregnancy come here. The women who need a hysterectomy or colposcopy come here, waiting alongside the women with a difficult menopause. The women who cannot conceive come here and sit watching other people carrying their newborn babies home. This is a building designed to arrange the obstetric and gynaecology services near each other. There is nowhere to breastfeed or pump here unless you are a postnatal inpatient, nowhere to make up a bottle. There are children everywhere but no playroom or creche. These days the café is run by a private company, not the volunteers who established it. The many community organisations that work with expectant families and parents with young babies are absent.

### COFFEE BREAK ACTIVITY

Draw a sketch of the layout of the waiting area in your antenatal clinic (hospital or community). Think about:
- What is the seating like?
- What is the signage like (Information? Instruction? Clear? Confusing? Stern? Friendly?)
- Is the area clean and uncluttered?

- What is the decoration like?
- Is it a noisy or quiet environment?
- What does it smell like?
- Are there toys or activities for children?
- Does it feel like a friendly calm place to you?

    We get very used to our own spaces including our working environments. Try to imagine what the forest of doors, signs and faces might feel like to someone who has never seen it before. How might they feel if they do not read English or are neurodiverse or uncertain if they want to be pregnant?

The NHS 15 Steps challenge—and the 15 Steps maternity toolkit (NHS England, 2018)—is a set of activities to observe and document how maternity services feel to service users.

> *Users of maternity services tell us their first impressions can make a huge difference to the confidence they feel. Therefore, teams should be reflecting upon whether the setting and staff are welcoming, friendly, informative, organised and calm.*
>
> (NHS ENGLAND, 2018, P. 10)

The intention is that within those first 15 steps into a new environment, service users will know how it makes them feel and whether they feel welcome and safe, or anxious, confused or overwhelmed. A key feature of the toolkit is to use service users as fresh eyes who can point out the things that we cannot see because we are so familiar. The maternity toolkit document recommends that service users drawn from minority groups are invaluable as fresh eyes because they are likely to feel more like outsiders and therefore any changes which work for them are likely also to be positive for the majority population.

## Continuing the Journey: Screening

The underlying theme of this next stop on our journey is uncertainty and complex decisions. Have a look at Chapter 5, Communicating Ideas, for discussion of complexity, uncertainty and risk across maternity care. In this section I ask a lot of questions. This is based on:

- **Key idea 3: By practice we get comfortable with uncertainty. We can then communicate in a more straightforward and calm manner.**

During perinatal care in the UK childbearing women and people will be offered screening from 6 of the 12 national population screening programmes (Office for Health Improvement and Disparities, 2022). They will therefore be making more screening decisions in a short space of time than they will over the rest of their lifetime.

Screening is about offering tests and follow-up care to people who are healthy and have no known signs or symptoms of the conditions the tests are about. It can be very hard for people to think about something that has so far not affected their life. Conversely, they may have very strong feelings because someone close to them, like a family member, has been affected by having or not having a screening test.

How we feel about screening as midwives is also informed by our personal experiences. If you or someone close to you has been affected by an antenatal screening decision, I want you to know strong feelings are totally normal. Please feel free to skip this section and come back to it when you are ready or not at all.

Most of the decisions a pregnant person must make are time sensitive and ideally made in very early pregnancy, but when they will have had little contact with midwifery services for support. It is important to communicate that screening programmes in the UK are a whole connected system which offers support with the conditions and anomalies identified. This is not the same in other countries, so pregnant women and people who are more familiar with other health care systems may have very different ideas about what to expect from their care.

Let's think about the concepts involved in making a decision about screening tests. First take a few minutes to reflect about your own learning about NHS antenatal and newborn screening programmes (ANNB). Try making some notes about the following questions.

**QUICK REFLECTION**

NHS antenatal and newborn screening programmes (ANNB).
- How difficult do you think the information is to process?
- How much do you think somebody needs to understand about a screening test to make a decision?
- How much do you think you personally need to understand about a test to recommend it?

National screening programmes in the UK are all based on looking for clear evidence that health care can improve outcomes if the condition is known about before signs and symptoms are present. Not all screening we offer has the same level of evidence of benefit, and you may need to convey information about how the screening programme was designed as well as the tests and treatments it offers. Antenatal screening may involve decisions about termination of a pregnancy, so when women or people have no intention to consider termination, they may still want to have screening for information.

Think now about the reality of a booking appointment in your practice. What are the most important things you and a pregnant woman or person need to communicate with each other, so that they can make a screening choice? How can you find out quickly what is important to them? How can you personalise your communication to support them?

Population screening programmes are designed on public health principles and so they are based on overall population and subgroup evidence. Guidance is based on judgements about what over time is likely to benefit the most people. A midwife's role in communicating about screening is to be an interpreter of something designed for everyone in a target population, into supporting an individual.

Like most areas of health care, screening programmes are subject to inverse care law. People who already experience social exclusion will experience exclusion and barriers during the screening programme—for example, they will be less likely to find out about it, be offered it, be less likely to accept it or be less likely to have successful follow-up (NHS England, 2021). Because the NHS screening programmes are based on the evidence and judgements that, ultimately, they will benefit most people, then reducing inequality strategies are based on encouraging more people to accept screening and in carrying it out successfully. You can do a lot to support equity in screening by improving your communication that is about access to the programme and follow-up.

Midwives take a central role in 1:1 or couple discussions about screening programmes. How will you communicate that screening can cause harms as well as offer potential benefits to an individual? How can we structure this communication without unduly triggering pregnant people's cognitive bias for risk aversion and support them to deal with uncertainty?

At this part of your journey with a pregnant woman or person you will probably not know each other very well. Even if you can offer them a continuity model of care you will still be in the initial stages of building trust and learning how to work together. In many cases you will be asking someone to process complex medical and ethical information on the first occasion you meet them.

Government information about screening communication focuses on the mechanics of communication—for example, considering language barriers and information available digitally or on paper (Office for Health Improvement and Disparities, 2022). This is fine as far as it goes but it doesn't tell us how our transmission of screening messages is heard and received (see Chapter 3). In this chapter I cannot offer you a template of how and what you should communicate with an individual pregnant woman or person, but I believe it helps to take time now to think-on-manual and do some 'meta-cognition'. Meta-cognition is thinking about our own thinking and our own feelings. How might you communicate these ideas:

- Rational versus gut feeling decision-making
- Benefit to most people versus benefits to me

- Tests based on certainty versus tests based on probability (for example, risk score calculations for Patau's syndrome versus detection of an infection, e.g., hepatitis)
- Does knowing make it possible to change something for the better? What does 'better' mean to me?
- Outcomes for the baby-to-be versus outcomes for the pregnant person
- Crossroads decisions—will this type of decision change how I live my life, and do I want that possibility (e.g., knowing you are HIV+)?
- Genetic conditions affect future pregnancy and your wider family (e.g., being a carrier for sickle cell disease)

There is very little research about what helps pregnant people make decisions about antenatal screening. A recent systematic review was commissioned by the government as part of the strategy to reduce inequalities in health care (Office for Health Improvement and Disparities, 2022). The review team considered research about improving access to screening but also about making decisions to accept it, where greater acceptance was a mark of greater equity. This brings us back into the circle of midwifery versus individual pregnant person 'positionality'. The review considered the rates of screening acceptance, but also at how well people understood information, and how happy they felt about the decision they had made.

Take a moment to do a little more meta-cognition here. What do you feel personally is most important to you? How might you find out what is most important to the person you are giving care to? If these judgements were different, what might you do?

Midwifery scholarship has been addressing the idea of 'informed choice' for decades, and there are interesting and complex debates across health care about balancing the ideas of being informed with being able to choose. The Health Disparity Review (2022) did not provide easy answers. Research that was reviewed tested short versus longer discussions and using video and written decision aids. Overall, the review did not find clear answers to what communication methods support pregnant women and people to make screening decisions. There was not enough research available to make firm recommendations (only four studies), and the most reliable research they found was too specific to give general answers about different groups of people or different types of decision.

There is one intriguing finding I'd like you to think about now. One study about structured decision support identified an inverse relationship between knowledge, satisfaction and uptake. This Health Disparity Review (2022) says this finding deserves more investigation but in the present we can only reflect on it. Remember this finding is not generalisable and the research was fairly old (1997). That said, how do you react to the idea that having greater understanding can cause us greater anxiety, less satisfaction with our decision and a greater chance we decline a test?

# Destinations: Birth Planning and Preferences

Pregnancy can be an intense and individual journey. Our final stop-off point brings us almost to our destination—the birth itself. This section briefly considers birth plans—what they can do, what they don't do, and how we can use them to have conversations around labour and birth.

**COFFEE BREAK ACTIVITY**

- What do you think a birth plan is for?
- How can it help/hinder communication between the labouring person and their caregiver?

The NHS has some overarching advice about birth plans on a webpage for families. It recommends that a birth plan is made and that it is a chance for people to express their wishes and preferences. However, it also reminds readers that 'You need to be flexible and prepared to do things differently from your birth plan if complications arise with you or your baby, or if facilities such as a birth pool aren't available' (NHS, 2021).

This suggests that whatever families may want, protocols and organisational factors are likely to take precedence.

**QUICK REFLECTION**

Think about a time you cared for someone with a detailed birth plan.
- Did you have a chance to discuss it with them?
- Was it easy to accommodate their wishes into your care?
- Did the care deviate from the plan and how did you manage this?

Birth plans have been around since birth moved into hospital in the late 1960s and became more widely recognised from the 1980s. They were initially a subversive tool written by women who were very aware of what the maternity services offered and wary of accepting it. This included procedures such as routine shaves and enemas, medications being given without clear consent and episiotomies regardless of clinical need. The value of written birth plans is unclear—a systematic review by Divall et al. (2016) found that there was no clear evidence to say that birth plans improved women's experiences or sense of control.

Midwives can also find birth plans challenging because they can lay bare the disconnect between what we think we are doing and what we are actually doing (Divall, 2018). We think we are providing person-centred individualised care, but our response to birth plans can be one of stress if they deviate from known pathways. We have seen in Chapter 8, Communication and Complex Care Planning, the importance of coming alongside women and families even when their wishes and plans go against our guidelines, protocols and ways of doing. In work on what women felt about birth plans, Divall et al. (2017) suggested that although they are a plank of late antenatal care in England, their value in their present form is not clear. They have moved from a woman-led tool to an array of templates and instructions issued by NHS Trusts and others. This rigid formulaic approach can make birth plans a tick-box exercise and reduces real communication and understanding between midwives and families. In their conclusion Divall et al. (2017) comment that:

> *Given findings from our own and others' studies, it may be that the phrase 'birth plan' is no longer appropriate for women and midwives, and it may be timely to reconsider terminology. Alternative ways in which women might express their labour and birth preferences should be determined and evaluated.*

As we can see from this quote, there is no such thing as the perfect birth plan, but every discussion comes back to open and honest communication. Look back to the case studies we talked about at the beginning of this chapter. Farhana has continued her pregnancy journey with you as her guide. At each appointment you have a chance to discuss her beliefs, hopes and anxieties—and those of Riz. This means that a birth plan may not seem necessary—you know her preferences and if you are caring for her in labour you can support her in order to make the experience as close to what she wants and needs as possible. In our more standard antenatal care pathway this may be more challenging, although it can still be possible to have conversations which build up to a picture of what someone wants from their labour and birth. Perhaps we need more flexibility in how we approach conversations—instead of a specific 'birth plan conversation' at 36 weeks, for example, we might have snippets of conversation through the pregnancy which help to build up that picture. Obviously with a different carer in labour it may be that these ideas need to be written down, but it may also be that with open and ongoing conversation pregnant people and their partners feel empowered to have conversations with their labour ward midwives rather than just hoping they read the completed birth plan template.

## Final Thoughts

Well here we are—we have reached our destination. As you can see, we have covered a lot of ground on our journey. I have stopped at specific points—booking, screening and birth plans to highlight some of the issues around communicating during the antenatal period. All of the ideas and principles can be applied to any pregnancy encounter or situation. The key is to keep that thinking switched to manual.

We also looked a bit more broadly at the landscape around us as we journeyed—equality, access, inclusion and the barriers to giving and receiving good quality communication.

I hope that you have enjoyed our travels and that they have given you some food for thought. Use this chapter in a way that works for you. It's been great meeting you and thank you for your company.

## References

Divall, B. (2018). Competing discourses of risk and woman-centred care: challenges for midwives and women. *International Journal of Birth and Parent Education*, 5(3).

Divall, B., Spiby, H., Roberts, J., & Walsh, D. (2016). Birth plans: A narrative review of the literature. *International Journal of Childbirth*, 6(3), 157–172. https://doi.org/10.1891/2156-5287.6.3.157.

Divall, B., Spiby, H., Nolan, M., & Slade, P. (2017). Plans, preferences or going with the flow: An online exploration of women's views and experiences of birth plans. *Midwifery*, 54, 29–34.

MBRRACE. (2021). MBRRACE-UK saving lives, improving mothers' care – Lessons learned to inform maternity care from the UK and Ireland Confidential Enquiries into Maternal Deaths and Morbidity 2017–19. https://www.npeu.ox.ac.uk/mbrrace-uk/reports

NHS England. The Fifteen Steps for Maternity – Quality from the perspective of people who use maternity services. 2018. https://www.england.nhs.uk/publication/the-fifteen-steps-for-maternity-quality-from-the-perspective-of-people-who-use-maternity-services/

NHS England. How to make a birth plan. 2021. https://www.nhs.uk/pregnancy/labour-and-birth/preparing-for-the-birth/how-to-make-a-birth-plan/

NHS England. (2021). NHS population screening: Identifying and reducing inequalities. https://www.gov.uk/guidance/nhs-population-screening-identifying-and-reducing-inequalities

NICE. (2021). Antenatal care guideline [NG201]. https://www.nice.org.uk/guidance/ng201

Ockenden, D. (2022). *Ockenden report – Final: findings, conclusions and essential actions from the independent review of maternity services at The Shrewsbury and Telford Hospital NHS Trust*. Her Majesty's Stationery Office (HMSO). [Online]. https://assets.publishing.service.gov.uk/government/uploads/system/uploads/attachment_data/file/1064302/Final-Ockenden-Report-web-accessible.pdf.

Office for Health Improvement and Disparities. *Population screening: review of interventions to improve participation among underserved groups*. 2022. UK Govt. https://www.gov.uk/government/publications/population-screening-improving-participation-in-underserved-groups/population-screening-review-of-interventions-to-improve-participation-among-underserved-groups

Office for Health Improvement and Disparities. *NHS screening programmes in England: 2019 to 2020*. 2022. https://www.gov.uk/government/publications/nhs-screening-programmes-annual-report/nhs-screening-programmes-in-england-2019-to-2020

## Resources

Public Health England Language Matters 2019. https://phescreening.blog.gov.uk/2019/06/04/language-matters-especially-if-youre-a-health-professional-talking-to-parents-to-be/
    *A useful page written by two parents of children looking at the use of inclusion language around screening and congenital abnormalities.*

Public Health England Summary animation and guidance 2021. https://www.gov.uk/government/publications/screening-tests-for-you-and-your-baby/introduction
    *Detailed information for the public—including video animations—looking at screening programmes in maternity.*

# CHAPTER 11

# Labour

Jo Gould

## Introduction

There is no doubt that childbirth can be a powerful and transformative event in women's lives. When things go right, women describe their births in terms such as feeling safe, strong, empowered and in control 'like a Goddess, or Queen'. Conversely, when things go wrong, women frequently describe their births in terms of failure, as terrifying, lonely and dehumanising. Surprisingly, these experiences are not necessarily correlated with physically traumatic experiences of birth. Risk of developing posttraumatic stress disorder (PTSD) following birth is strongly associated with interpersonal/communication difficulties with caregivers (Harris & Ayers, 2012). Communication between health care professionals and women during labour and birth has a profound impact on the experience. This is magnified in the midwife–mother relationship, where sensitive communication is the foundation from which a relationship of trust is built. Continuity and relational models of care can make this task easier, but in settings where the midwife is not known to the woman in advance of labour, good communication skills to build trust rapidly and effectively are vital. With all this in mind, this chapter aims to provide a detailed exploration of communication in relation to labour, birth and the immediate postnatal period. Compassionate communication in early labour via telephone triage will be considered. Responsive verbal and nonverbal communication in established labour, birth and the immediate postnatal period will be explored. Communication and informed consent will be discussed. Finally, the chapter will consider communication related to information exchange, handover and record keeping.

## Telephone Triage and Compassionate Communication in Early Labour

The very first point of contact between a woman in labour and her care provider is typically via a maternity telephone triage system. Telephone triage is an effective way of sifting and sorting the assessment, appropriate advice and ongoing care of women who use the maternity services from an organisational perspective. From the perspective of a service user, telephone communication in early labour via triage has the capacity to set the scene for everything that follows. In other words, it has huge potential to impact on the woman's experience of care overall. One of the problems with all interactions in labour is the disparity of experience between the midwife and the labouring woman. A single midwife working in a triage unit will assess a significant number of women via a telephone conversation in a typical day and more than a hundred women in a typical month. A woman in labour may have this experience just once or twice in a lifetime. The triage midwife has the advantage of being in a familiar environment, in a familiar team, doing things that are routinely part of their work role, that they may do day in, day out. The woman in early labour finds herself in very unfamiliar territory. She may be at home but is likely to be experiencing the new and frightening sensations of labour. She may be in the presence of a birth partner, someone who is providing support to the best of their ability but who is also extremely uncertain about the situation. Unless the woman is planning a homebirth, she will be aware that at some point she will need to get into a car and journey to a birth centre or obstetric unit. The fear that their baby will be born en route to the birth centre or obstetric unit is nearly always present. The situation therefore has the potential to be fraught with fear and uncertainty. A telephone call to the maternity unit and a midwife who sounds overly busy and business-like in nature is enough to add to this. It may be challenging for a triage midwife to come to every telephone conversation and respond with empathy when it is such a routine part of the job; the practice environment is often a busy and stressful one and the assessment must be made quickly and efficiently. But a midwife's ability to communicate with compassion at this point has the capacity to bridge the disparity of experience between herself and the mother and to alleviate some of the fear and uncertainty that typifies women's experiences of early labour. This is at least as important as taking a full history from the woman. Good communication starts with the very first interaction between the mother and the maternity unit and has the potential to last a lifetime.

The way to overcome much of this is to tip the balance of care much more in favour of the woman and family and avoid hospital-based telephone triage systems altogether. Central to the vision of 'Better births' (NHS, 2016) are relational continuity models of care. These models have the potential to avoid some of the issues presented by large-scale triage systems, by restoring a more human and personalised interaction between the woman and her midwife. However, until relational continuity is fully realised, it is worth exploring how communication via telephone triage may be used not just as an assessment tool for the midwife but as a tool to alleviate some of the fear and uncertainty associated with women's experiences of early labour and birth.

If compassion is defined as 'sympathetic pity and concern for the sufferings or misfortunes of others' (Cambridge English Dictionary, 2022), then compassionate communication should reflect this. This can be challenging when communicating over the phone. Active listening is a technique that is widely used in counselling and therapy, and its roots can be traced to Carl Rogers, one of the founding fathers of psychotherapy. Three key elements are present in active listening; the first is the communication of nonverbal involvement, or the sense of giving the labouring woman unconditional attention. Over the telephone, this means listening attentively and agreeing with a 'yes', or 'mmm hmm'. This feedback will help the woman to feel more at ease and more comfortable to continue speaking. The second is the use of paraphrasing, or 'restating' what the labouring woman has communicated (both content AND feelings), in other words, mirroring the woman's story of her labour. Finally, encourage the woman to elaborate on her feelings. Be patient and avoid interrupting or speaking over the woman. The tendency to interrupt and lead the conversation often reflects the busy practice environment. The midwife may be able to assess what has been happening physically to the woman, but the impact on her, of not *really* being heard, is significant. Be aware that there will be natural pauses which do not need to be filled with speech; try to listen and wait for the woman to continue. These responses build empathy and trust by demonstrating an understanding of the woman's experience that is being described, without judgement. The midwife can take a full history from the woman via active listening *and* enable the woman to feel heard and understood. Both are achieved through effective communication and are the foundation of high-quality care in early labour.

### QUICK REFLECTION

Think about a time when you had to speak to someone in a call centre about something that was important to you. Or perhaps a time when you had to call to discuss a sensitive issue with your GP surgery and you had to negotiate the appointment with an unsupportive receptionist. Make a note of how you felt when the person you spoke to appeared to be too busy/unresponsive/uninterested to help you or trotted out the 'party line'.

Conversely, think of a time when someone in this situation came across in a particularly human way. What did they say or do that stands out?

Now reflect upon your own practice as a midwife communicating with women in early labour over the phone. Can you see any similarities or limitations associated with this? Consider the following questions:

1. How might the way in which you communicate be received by someone feeling vulnerable?
2. How does the working environment impact on this?
3. Is there anything that you can alter in either of these areas to improve early labour communication over the telephone?

Three key practice/learning points:

- Use the woman's name throughout the telephone call and state your own name and availability for further calls. This is a very simple act and easily overlooked, but one which is immediately more human and personal. The sense that there is someone familiar to interact starts to build trust between the woman and her caregivers. Don't forget to introduce yourself to the birth partner (who is likely to make the first contact) *and* the labouring woman, when you start to speak to her.
- Try to maintain awareness of the disparity of experience between yourself and the labouring woman. Remain attuned to the sense of vulnerability that women feel when experiencing early labour. Avoid professional jargon and language that is disempowering; plain English enhances connection between the woman and the midwife taking the call.
- Cultivate active listening skills and provide positive feedback on the woman's progress so far. Fully explain the rationale for advising the woman to stay at home, if that is your assessment and recommendation. Women frequently report feeling that they didn't understand why they were made to stay at home without midwifery support in early labour. Clear explanations and advice regarding coping strategies and further contact as and when required make a huge difference.

Three ideas to take into practice:

- Have a look at the Nursing and Midwifery Council publication *Standards of Proficiency for Midwives* (NMC, 2019). Domain 6 sets out the breadth of midwifery skills situated in the five domains of proficiency. Communication is an overarching skill across all domains. Find domain 6.1 and consider the detailed communication skills set out in relation to your own experience of telephone triage. Web link: https://www.nmc.org.uk/globalassets/sitedocuments/standards/standards-of-proficiency-for-midwives.pdf
- Develop self-awareness skills via the 360-degree feedback form provided later in the chapter. Give to five close friends and/or colleagues to complete and return to you. Developing greater insight into how others see you is a brilliant starting point for improving your self-awareness in relation to the women and families you care for (360-degree feedback activity University Hospitals Birmingham,2021).
- One of the limitations of telephone triage is the lack of face-to-face contact. A quality, service improvement and redesign project (QSIR) (NHS England, 2021a) focused on the use of digital/video consultation for triage might be a good way to improve this. Face-to-face contact with another person, even via a video call, has the potential to alleviate some of the 'faceless' nature of telephone triage and supports the relationship building and trust that is so important for women's psychological safety in labour.

## Communication and Attunement During Established Labour and Birth

Building a trusting relationship with women for labour and birth begins with the first communication in early labour via telephone and continues when the woman is in established labour and being cared for in person. The use of active listening techniques throughout established labour and birth (described earlier) will continue to develop an atmosphere of empathy and trust. The advantage of being face to face means the midwife can use nonverbal skills to help the woman to feel more at ease. Welcoming the woman on arrival, introducing yourself fully and smiling genuinely are small acts but make a huge difference to someone arriving at an unfamiliar labour ward or birth centre. At homebirth, this initial interaction is equally important. As physiological labour advances and becomes more intense, the woman becomes more tired and more vulnerable. Sensitive and responsive communication techniques, verbal and nonverbal, on the part of the midwife can help to mitigate the woman's sense of vulnerability and provide support. Conversely, insensitive communication can increase the woman's sense of vulnerability. Chatting to other staff, speaking loudly or during contractions are examples of insensitive practices that are not received well by women in labour. These behaviours model a degree of not really understanding or caring about the extreme nature of what the woman is experiencing. To reiterate an earlier point: issues with the interpersonal skills of the care provider during labour and birth are the strongest predictor of PTSD. In one study the communication skills of the health care professionals were cited as the largest cause of postbirth PTSD (Harris & Ayers, 2012).

There is a beautiful description of sensitive and responsive communication in a recent qualitative study focused on midwives supporting women's alternative birth choices in the NHS (Feeley et al., 2022). The term 'attunement' describes the way in which an experienced midwife uses sensitive communication to harmonise with a woman in labour, to go to where she is:

> You just, you just ... talk nicely to people and you go to that place where they are rather than expecting them to somehow meet you ... on your plane, it's theirs, it's their space it's their experience and you go to where they are ... you go in and you put yourself in that space, you talk softer and you respond less, you respond to make them feel ... comfortable.

> (FEELEY ET AL., 2022).

In essence, this quote from the research demonstrates the midwife's ability to communicate with empathy; they tune into the woman's experience and respond accordingly. The midwife views the labour space as the woman's and responds with sensitivity, speaking softly and responding to the woman, rather than leading. This expertise—the ability to watch, listen and respond with all senses—is at the heart of expert midwifery practice. Leap (2010) describes how hard it is, when a midwife is 'thrown' together with a woman in labour, to not talk too much, or tell jokes or do *too* much try and build rapport and trust. Although this isn't bad practice, it is the opposite of attunement, it does not try to *really* go to where the woman is.

Several women in Tricia Anderson's seminal study on women's experiences of the second stage of labour describe in powerful terms their awareness of the midwife and what she was doing and/or saying at a point when they felt ultimately vulnerable (Anderson, 2010). The midwife, when trusted by the labouring woman, is described as an anchor, someone who helps the woman to feel safer. At this point, the midwife is in an extraordinarily powerful position, because the woman is at the peak of her vulnerability. She is tired, and may have been in pain for many hours, possibly even days. She may feel extremely out of control. Several of the study participants at this intense stage of labour described feeling as though they had entered an altered state of consciousness, which is a primitive survival technique. The women described out-of-body experiences, feeling the loss of control of their bodies and loss of normal consciousness, time distortion and loss of awareness of the room. Despite this altered consciousness, many women described being tuned into what the midwife was doing or saying. Altered consciousness is linked to the low-frequency theta and delta brainwaves seen via encephalograms (EEGs). Theta brainwaves are associated with daydreaming, light sleep and deep hypnosis. This brain activity is believed to play an important part in processing information and making memories. This altered state of consciousness has been linked to the potential to develop PTSD when perceptions of labour and birth care are negative (Harris & Ayers, 2012). Sensitive and supportive communication at this point is therefore of critical importance. Rhiannon, one of the mothers in Anderson's study, describes perfectly the power of the midwife in the second stage of labour:

> *You're at the most vulnerable point because you can't do anything. If someone starts telling you to do something, you just do it. When the midwife told me that I wasn't to push or to do something—like turn over—I felt like a little schoolgirl: 'Oh alright then—if I have to'. So midwives are in a real position of power which they mustn't abuse.*
> (RHIANNON QUOTED IN ANDERSON, 2010)

This description links to another critical component at the heart of communication in labour, which is power relationships. As described by Rhiannon, from the mother's perspective the power of the midwife during labour and birth is enormous. Describing herself as feeling 'like a little schoolgirl' links to Berne's transactional analysis theory (Berne, 1957). It is useful to summarise Berne's theory here, because even a basic understanding will help develop better awareness of the negative potential of power relationships when communicating during labour and birth.

Transactional analysis was founded by Eric Berne in the 1950s and was influenced by Freud's theory of psychoanalysis, which centres on the potential for childhood experiences to shape adult life (Berne, 1957). Berne proposed that the human personality is made up of three ego states: parent, adult and child. The ego states are systems of thought, feeling and behaviour. The ego states underpin all social interactions and are influenced by childhood experiences (including trauma), context and by other people's behaviour/ego states. Rhiannon's quote demonstrates how easy it is for women to slip into the child ego state during labour and birth when presented with a midwife communicating in a particularly directive style. This is a fundamental learning point when it comes to communication. Anything that increases a woman's sense of vulnerability and effectively disempowers her should be avoided. In addition, for survivors of childhood sexual abuse (CSA) the trotting out of orders to push or not push, change position or not, and so on, has enormous potential for triggering trauma. That's not to say that the midwife doesn't ever need to ask the woman to do any of this, it just means that the way such requests are communicated is of great importance (see points to take into practice, later).

Similarly, the use of nonverbal communication has great potential to increase the sense of vulnerability felt by women in labour. The NMC Standards for Proficiency (2019) set out specific expectations for both verbal and nonverbal communication, prioritising eye contact, touch and respecting personal space. Something as simple as how the midwife positions themselves in relation to the woman is of great importance. A routine occurrence on busy labour wards, where midwives and other health care professionals feel comfortable, or 'on their turf', is the tendency to stand over a woman on a bed and talk 'down' to her. The obstetrician Marsden Wagner identified that health care professionals working in maternity develop a very specific culture of working and because they are so immersed in this culture, day in, day out, they can't see the good and bad parts anymore. His description of this was 'fish can't see water'. To avoid losing awareness of poor communication practices, maintaining self-awareness and developing positive 'rituals' when it comes to verbal and nonverbal communication are key. The bed example earlier is easily remedied by the midwife paying conscious attention to how they position themselves in relation to the woman when communicating. Alongside, at eye level (or preferably below) places the woman above the midwife, which will help her to feel much less vulnerable. The appropriate use of touch, a hand on the woman's hand, for example, can also be reassuring. This is a hard skill to learn, and it is worth paying attention to how practice supervisors and colleagues navigate the use of touch when caring for women in labour. An obstetrician I worked with many years ago as a student midwife was an expert in reassuring nonverbal communication. No matter what the situation, he would draw up a low stool and sit alongside the woman, always slightly lower than her when quietly communicating difficult information, always with great sensitivity, occasionally placing a well-judged hand on her hand. It was a powerful exercise in how to diminish the woman's sense of vulnerability at a stressful point in labour.

Three key practice/learning points:

- If you have worked in both the hospital and community setting, reflect on the differences between caring for someone in labour at home and in hospital. Think about the verbal and nonverbal communication that decreases women's sense of vulnerability, described earlier. Are there differences in the two settings? If so, how can you replicate the positive examples in all birth settings?
- Read the chapter 'Feeling Safe Enough to Let Go' in *The Midwife Mother Relationship* (Anderson, 2010) to gain greater insight into the vulnerability women feel in the second stage of labour. Think about how the midwife's communication at this point is received by the woman.
- Maintaining good self-awareness is the key to maintaining empathic communication when caring for women during labour and birth and is one of the four pillars of emotional intelligence. Try completing this questionnaire to gain more insight into your own self-awareness: https://www.mindtools.com/pages/article/ei-quiz.htm

Three ideas to take into practice:

- When working on the labour ward (on a rare quiet day!), encourage colleagues to try out the lithotomy position and take turns to experience how this feels. Try 'talking down' to the person lying on the bed. Conversely, try sitting alongside the person and talking to them. Reflect as a team on common feelings/themes from the exercise. Is this exercise something you could write up and present in your local area? Think about involving the local Maternity Voices Partnership (MVP) in the process too. Connecting with service users and working together to improve communication will result in better experiences for women and families. Involve the head of midwifery, obstetric and education teams with this exercise.
- When you next look after a woman in normal labour, try to 'go to where the woman is'. Tune in to her experience and respond to her cues throughout the process, rather than lead conversations or fill in gaps with small talk. Reflect upon how that feels. It is a good way to develop responsive communication skills.
- Reflect upon time spent as a student midwife witnessing the way in which your mentor communicated with women and families. Does anything stand out, positive or negative? Think about your own communication style and try to identify the strengths and areas for development.

## Communication in the Immediate Postbirth Period

There is very little published evidence to inform midwives regarding communication in the immediate postbirth period, which is often referred to as 'the golden hour'. This concept has been adopted from adult emergency medicine. Here, the first hour after traumatic injury and the subsequent management determine survival of the patient. In the first hour postbirth the mother and the baby are both making huge physiological transitions. For the mother, the birth of the placenta marks the start of the return to a nonpregnant physiological state and the initiation of lactation. For the baby, the transition is from intrauterine to extrauterine life. Unrestricted skin-to-skin contact between the mother and baby supports these physiological transitions, optimises oxytocin release in preparation for breastfeeding and bonding, and inhibits stress responses in both mother and baby (Buckley & Uvnas-Moberg, 2019). This time is critical in facilitating the process of attachment between the woman and her baby and her transition to the role of mother. The behaviour and communication skills of the midwife can support or inhibit these processes.

A small qualitative study in Finland confirmed what is commonly seen in maternity units in the UK: the needs of the institution overshadow the needs of the woman, baby and family at this critical point in their lives (Niela-Vilen et al., 2020). The study found that midwives were very much in control of the postbirth period, following guidelines and performing activities, such as managing the delivery of the placenta, newborn checks, weighing, vitamin K administration and so on. Time pressures almost certainly exacerbate this efficient behaviour. The researchers identified the embedded power of the midwives which encouraged parents to comply with their needs, rather than voice their own. Power and vulnerability have been discussed in relation to how midwives communicate earlier in the chapter, and both have great relevance in the immediate postnatal period. At this time, women are through the majority of the birth process and simultaneously relieved and delighted to finally meet their babies. For first-time mothers, vulnerability takes on a new form, that of feeling like an absolute novice in respect of the status of mother that has been immediately thrust upon them by the birth. This is momentous and the start of the long transition from woman to mother. The midwife and the way in which she facilitates and communicates during this time have a potentially powerful and long-lasting impact.

Prioritising a warm, quiet, calm environment and facilitating skin-to-skin contact between mother and baby optimise the neurohormonal activity that optimises physiology. For the mother, this will support the birth of the placenta and subsequent haemostasis; for the baby, this will support the stabilisation of heart rate, respiration and temperature. In line with this, communication should be responsive and calm. If all is well, the communication should be mother led, with the midwife responding. The woman is likely to ask questions about the placenta, about the baby, about starting to breastfeed. The midwife should try to respond to the mother's cues, rather than 'leading'. The specific needs of each individual are more likely to be met in this way. Positive feedback at this point is powerful. First-time mothers feel their lack of experience and knowledge, and positive feedback in relation to their interactions with their babies starts to develop their identity and ability as mothers. Using communication that acknowledges any feelings of 'not knowing', followed by reassurances of mothers becoming experts in their own babies in no time at all, will be reassuring. The 'tasks' required following this undisturbed skin-to-skin contact and first feed can be introduced sensitively, using language such as 'Would it be ok to …' or 'When would you like me to …' rather than 'I need to …' or 'I have to …'. It is a small difference but demonstrates respect for the mother in relation to her baby and rebalances the power dynamic described previously, giving more to the woman. These actions are sensitive and respectful to the needs of the woman and the baby at this point, which is critical in terms of psychological safety and ongoing transition to motherhood. The woman, her partner and family's involvement in the 'tasks' is a good way to promote interactive communication. At this point, the midwife should communicate carefully regarding the interventions that are being offered, including the relevant evidence and rationale, before gaining consent. This should be tailored to each family and will facilitate the start of getting to know their baby 'on the outside'.

Three key practice/learning points:

- Prioritise a calm, quiet environment immediately postbirth. Think about how this can be achieved in all practice environments. Facilitate mother-led, rather than midwife-led, communication as much as possible.
- When carrying out the 'tasks' associated with this immediate postbirth period, use respectful language that seeks permission from parents, rather than dictating what needs to be done from the midwife perspective. Involve the parents as much as possible with these tasks and offer explanation and information. This is reassuring for the parents and helps to start the process of helping them to become knowledgeable and responsive to their baby's needs.
- Remember that positive feedback at this point facilitates the transition the mother is starting to make to becoming 'expert' in her role and relationship with her baby.

## Informed Consent in Labour and Birth

The principle of informed consent is embedded in modern health care. Its use in maternity has been under the microscope since the legal case 'Montgomery vs Lanarkshire' was decided in the UK Supreme Court in 2015. The case was brought by Nadine Montgomery, a woman with diabetes who experienced a shoulder dystocia during her son's birth which resulted in his cerebral palsy. She was not told of the risk of this complication occurring during vaginal birth, despite questioning whether the size of her baby was likely to cause problems. The court found in Montgomery's favour and established new standards for informed consent, which were much more patient focused. Health care professionals are now expected to fully discuss the material risks of clinical procedures and processes with patients to ensure informed consent for these has been given. The Montgomery ruling was reinforced by the interim findings of the Ockenden report, produced following the review of Shrewsbury and Telford maternity services (Ockenden, 2020). Repeated failures of care over many years were investigated and seven immediate and essential actions were identified for all maternity units in England to implement. One of these action points is improvement to informed consent:

> *All maternity services must ensure the provision to women of accurate and contemporaneous evidence-based information as per national guidance. This must include all aspects of maternity care throughout the antenatal, intrapartum and postnatal periods of care.*
>
> (OCKENDEN, 2020)

In addition, domain 1 'Prioritising People' in the NMC Code (2018) reinforces the need for midwives to work in partnership with women and families, involving them in decisions about their care and respecting and documenting their right to accept or refuse treatment.

For midwives caring for women during established labour and birth, there are challenges to obtaining informed consent. Women in advanced labour may find it more difficult to absorb information regarding the relative risks and benefits of interventions. The midwife needs to take care over this, because the impact of not providing enough information for the woman to make a truly informed choice results in increased vulnerability to legal action at some point further down the line. For women, there are two major consequences. One is the situation Nadine Montgomery found herself in, having important information withheld from her which had devastating consequences for her son. The other consequence, and arguably far more common, is the lack of a complete picture regarding the risks of interventions. Postbirth, women start to question how their labours ended up taking a particular turn. A study examining the use of decision aids to support informed decision-making in obstetrics found that women often expressed 'decision regret' at accepting interventions, because they did not understand the impact they would have upon their labours (Vlemmix et al., 2013). Typical examples of poorly informed and consented procedures include induction of labour, artificial rupture of the membranes and oxytocin augmentation. By providing fully informed choice and consent during the process of labour and birth, the midwife can address these issues. Ideally, typical examples of labour and birth interventions should be fully discussed and documented during pregnancy and ahead of labour, when women can consider information without the added stress of being tired and in pain. Rechecking consent in labour is then a quicker and easier process. Either way, there is a useful decision-making tool, BRAIN (see the following case study), that can be used quickly and effectively to ensure that informed consent for routine labour interventions has been given. Consideration needs to be given to developing clear communication strategies for non-English speakers. Use of telephone language services, interpreter services and translation devices should be made to ensure equal access to high-quality information. The midwife must also check understanding following discussions related to interventions. The simplest way to do this is to ask the woman to repeat and describe what she understands by what has been communicated. Communication is a two-way process; it is not good enough to simply 'give' information without checking understanding. Gaps and/or issues with understanding can then be addressed by the midwife until sure that the woman fully understands before consent is given and documented.

## Case Study

### Informed Choice and Consent in Labour (Using the BRAIN Tool)

Charlotte is a G2, P0, 40+2. Her pregnancy has been healthy and straightforward with a well-grown baby. Charlotte had a previous spontaneous vaginal delivery and is booked for a homebirth this time. She is admitted to the labour ward via triage following spontaneous rupture of membranes at 0220 hours, with thick fresh meconium. She is contracting strongly, 1:3, feeling anxious about the meconium, stressed about being in hospital and uncertain about what happens next. The midwife allocated to her needs has to discuss the hospital protocol of continuous electronic foetal monitoring (CEFM, which is recommended when thick meconium liquor is present) and gain informed consent for this procedure. The BRAIN tool is a useful acronym for the midwife to base this discussion on. This will give Charlotte a full picture of the intervention that is being offered to her, increasing the likelihood of fully informed consent being given. In relation to cardiotocograph (CTG) in the presence of thick meconium liquor, a BRAIN discussion might go something like this:

**Benefits:** For a small number of babies, thick meconium liquor can indicate that there may have been some issues with oxygenation for the baby in response to labour. It isn't possible to identify affected babies and so CTG monitoring is recommended in all cases of thick meconium liquor, to identify affected babies and improve outcomes. Affected babies are at higher risk of inhaling the thick meconium into their lungs around the time of birth, making breathing and oxygenation extremely challenging for them.

**Risks:** The evidence for CTG monitoring is poor. It increases the risk of interventions, such as instrumental birth and emergency Caesarean section with conflicting evidence of improved outcomes. In addition, it limits mobility in labour, which makes the process more challenging to manage without epidural anaesthesia.

**Alternatives:** Listening to the baby's heartbeat with a handheld device, such as a Sonic aid. This would not be recommended as it is not possible to produce a continuous 'picture' of the baby's heart rate using this method.

**Intuition:** What is Charlotte's gut feeling about the offer of CTG monitoring? This is important, and strong gut feelings about what is right for the woman are underpinned by her culture and beliefs and must be respected by the midwife, in line with the NMC Code (2018).

**Nothing:** Or the option to do nothing. If there is no monitoring, it is very difficult to assess how the baby is managing throughout the process of labour and this is of particular concern due to the thick meconium liquor. Affected babies are more likely to be admitted and treated in a special care baby unit (SCBU)/neonatal intensive care unit (NICU).

The BRAIN conversation will enable Charlotte to make a quick, but fully informed decision regarding the offer of CTG monitoring and the midwife can be sure that truly informed consent has been given before proceeding.

Three key practice/learning points:

- Get into the habit of using the BRAIN acronym when discussing labour and birth interventions.
- Ensure high-quality communication of information is facilitated for non-English speakers via the use of interpreters and translation devices and tools such as telephone language services. Avoid using family members for translation wherever possible.
- Check the woman's understanding of interventions being offered by asking her to describe what she has been told.

Ideas to take into practice:

- Investigate your maternity unit's resources for service users where English is not their first language. Consider how these might be used in relation to high-quality informed decision-making and consent. If you identify gaps, think about how these could be addressed. Seek support from your head of midwifery, governance leads, maternity safety and quality committee and local Maternity Voices Partnership.

## Information Exchange, Handover and Documentation

The way in which health care professionals engage in communication during the handover of care has a direct impact on outcomes. Poor communication is cited as a component in the maternal deaths reported in successive MBRRACE-UK (Mothers and Babies: Reducing Risk Through Audits and Confidential Enquiries Across the UK) enquiries. In busy, fast-moving environments, such as labour wards, it is relatively easy to miss passing on significant information during the handover of care. Systematic handover tools, such as SBAR (situation, background, assessment, recommendations) or CHAPS (clinical picture, history, assessment, plan), are in widespread use and can support the midwife in ensuring that significant information regarding women in their care is accurately and effectively communicated to colleagues.

SBAR was developed via the US Military for communication on nuclear submarines. It has been adapted for use in health care as part of the drive to improve patient safety (NHS England, 2021a, 2021b). Standardised prompts are used to enable staff to communicate concise, focused information, reducing omissions, repetition and the likelihood of errors. Use of SBAR in maternity encourages staff to engage in a standardised approach to handover, with a consistent level of detail (see the following box for an example of maternity SBAR tool).

Situation
• Reason for admission or transfer
• Gestation
• Parity
• High/low risk

Background
• Obstetric history
• Medical history
• Reason for admission
• Clinical picture
• Rhesus status
• Medication/allergies

Assessment
• Clinical history
• Observations
• Examinations
• Partogram/labour progress
• Pain relief
• Blood loss
• Spontaneous rupture of membranes (SROM)

Recommendations
• Plan of care

Handover from:

Handover to:

Date & time:

Adapted from Spranzi and Norton (2020).

# Documentation

The chapter so far has focused on aspects of verbal and nonverbal communication. Written communication skills are of equal importance, because of the need to fully document the care that is given. The requirement for midwives to keep clear and accurate records in relation to their practice is set out in the NMC Code (2018). The documentation of care should be completed at the time the care is delivered, or as soon as possible afterwards. Late entries should be noted as such, for example, noted as 'Recorded in retrospect', timed, dated and signed by the person making the entry. All entries should be accurately recorded, not falsified, written clearly without the use of unnecessary jargon or abbreviation, and signed, timed and dated. Maternity is one of the most common NHS specialities for litigation and records kept by midwives can be used as evidence in legal action in future. Documentation of care given is essentially evidence of that care. Therefore all relevant information should be recorded. This is increasingly occurring via electronic records and the same principles apply to both written and digital records. In all cases, it is the responsibility of the midwife to ensure records are kept securely.

Three key practice/learning points:

- Tools that have been developed for systematic handover of care between health care professionals improve patient safety.
- Reflect upon the handover of care in your practice area and between different health care professionals. Are there differences in the way different professionals communicate? Note down the positives and negatives and be aware of these the next time you need to do a handover.
- Try to involve women and families in the handover of care, from midwife to midwife, or midwife to obstetrician whenever possible. This will create an open and honest environment for communication and will increase the sense of trust between the woman, partner, family and health care team. In addition, it gives the woman a further opportunity to develop better understanding of her situation and care being delivered.

Three ideas to take into practice:

- How are handovers of care conducted in your own area of practice? Are they always effective? If not, what are the barriers to this and can they be mitigated? Noisy and distracting environments are a good example of this, and moving to a quieter area for handover makes an enormous difference.
- Is there a handover tool in use in your own area of practice? If not, speak to your Head of Midwifery, Quality and Safety Committee or education team about implementing a more systematic approach, using SBAR, or similar. If there is a handover tool in use, is it always used effectively? This would be a good area to investigate via an audit and improve the effectiveness of handovers of care.
- If you are a student midwife, during a quieter shift, practise using the SBAR handover tool discussed earlier to summarise the key points from a case that you are involved with and present to your practice supervisor. This will help you to develop the skills required to meet the communication proficiencies in your practice assessment documents.

# Conclusion

The use of communication as a tool to alleviate some of the fear and uncertainty associated with women's experiences of early labour and birth is as important as the communication used to make assessments of labour progress and subsequent admission to the birth centre or maternity unit. It may feel even more important to women.

Sensitive and responsive verbal and nonverbal communication during labour, birth and the immediate postnatal period has a transformative and potentially lifelong impact on women's experiences. Poor communication during this time is strongly correlated with PTSD.

The case to strengthen the way in which informed choice and consent are communicated during labour and birth has been identified in this chapter. It is important for the midwife from a legal perspective, and for the mother's understanding and decision-making. This has a significant impact on the long-term wellbeing of the mother when she processes her birth experience. In addition, in situations where there are language barriers, assistance must be given to obtain informed consent via the clearest possible communication via translation tools and interpreter services wherever possible.

## References

Anderson, T. (2010). Felling safe enough to let go: The relationship between a woman and her midwife during the second stage of labour. In Kirkham, M. (Ed.), *The midwife mother relationship* (2nd ed.). Palgrave Macmillan.

Berne, E. (1957). Ego states in psychotherapy. *American Journal of Psychotherapy*, *11*(2), 293–309.

Buckley, S., & Uvnas-Moberg, K. (2019). Nature and consequences of oxytocin and other neuro-hormones during the perinatal period. In Downe, S., & Byrom, S. (Eds.), *Squaring the circle*. Pinter & Martin.

Cambridge English Dictionary. (2022). *Compassion*. https://dictionary.cambridge.org/dictionary/english/compassion. Accessed 24 February 2022.

Feeley, C., Downe, S., & Thompson, G. (2022). 'Stories of distress versus fulfilment': A narrative inquiry of midwives' experiences supporting alternative birth choices in the UK National Health Service. *Women & Birth*, *35*, e446–e445.

Harris, R., & Ayers, S. (2012). What makes labour and birth traumatic? A survey of intrapartum hotspots. *Psychology & Health*, *27*(10), 1166–1177.

Leap, N. (2010). The less we do, the more we give. In Kirkham, M. (Ed.), *The midwife mother relationship* (2nd ed.). Palgrave Macmillan.

Ockenden, D. (2020). Emerging findings and recommendations from the independent review of maternity services at the Shrewsbury and Telford Hospital NHS Trust. https://assets.publishing.service.gov.uk/government/uploads/system/uploads/attachment_data/file/943011/Independent_review_of_maternity_services_at_Shrewsbury_and_Telford_Hospital_NHS_Trust.pdf. Accessed 24 February 2022.

NHS England. (2016). *Better births. Improving outcomes of maternity services in England, a five year forward view for maternity care.* NHS England.

NHS England. (2021a). *Quality, service improvement and redesign tools.* https://www.england.nhs.uk/sustainableimprovement/qsir-programme/qsir-tools/. Accessed 24 February 2022.

NHS England. (2021b). *Online library of quality, service improvement and redesign tools. SBAR communication tool—Situation, background, assessment, recommendation.* https://www.england.nhs.uk/wp-content/uploads/2021/03/qsir-sbar-communication-tool.pdf. Accessed 24 February 2022.

Niela-Vilen, H., Axelin, A., & Flacking, R. (2020). The golden hour in Finnish birthing units—An Ethnographic study. *Midwifery, 89*, 102793. https://doi.org/10.1016/j.midw.2020.102793.

Nursing & Midwifery Council. (2018). *The code. Professional standards of practice and behaviour for nurses, midwives and nursing associates.* https://www.nmc.org.uk/globalassets/sitedocuments/nmc-publications/nmc-code.pdf. Accessed 24 February 2022.

Nursing & Midwifery Council. (2019). *Standards of proficiency for midwives.* https://www.nmc.org.uk/globalassets/sitedocuments/standards/standards-of-proficiency-for-midwives.pdf. Accessed 24 February 2022.

Spranzi, F., & Norton, C. (2020). From handover to takeover: Should we consider a new conceptual model of communication? *British Journal of Midwifery, 28*(3), 156–165.

The Supreme Court. (2015). Montgomery (Appellant) v Lanarkshire Health Board (Respondent) (Scotland). https://www.supremecourt.uk/cases/docs/uksc-2013-0136-judgment.pdf. Accessed 24 February 2022.

Vlemmix, F., Warendorf, J., Rosman, A., Kok, M., Mol, B., Morris, J., & Nassar, N. (2013). Decision aids to improve informed decision-making in pregnancy care: A systematic review. *British Journal of Obstetrics & Gynaecology, 120*(3), 257–266.

## Resources

University Hospitals Birmingham (2021). 360-degree feedback. https://www.uhb.nhs.uk/education/career-development/appraisals/360-degree-feedback.htm
*Use this feedback form to think about your practice, and how you come across to others.*

# CHAPTER 12

# The Postnatal Period and Infant Feeding

Michelle Tant

## Introduction

The postnatal period is a time of significant adjustment in the woman or other birthing person's life. They will need to navigate the physiological changes as well as the psychological and emotional journey of becoming parents. Each will have their own unique experience relating to background, culture and spiritual beliefs, but there are some universally experienced characteristics which transport them to a worldwide connectivity with others who have newly given birth. However, these factors may well also have an impact on the person's experience of those feelings.

Women and other birthing people are being communicated with continually from all angles. Midwives need to be able to acknowledge these complexities and competing narratives, plus the pressures placed on women and birthing people to meet unrealistic expectations in this vulnerable period of transition. They are ideally placed to communicate openly and honestly with women and birthing people about the physical, psychological and emotional aspects of the postnatal period and must be adequately prepared to do so. Therefore in this chapter we will be discussing some of the pressures on new parents to meet unrealistic expectations of the postpartum body about infant feeding and consider what role midwives have in bringing balance to this conversation. Finally, we will consider the emotional and psychological transition to parenthood and the impact of birth trauma which serves to further reduce the 'bandwidth' of new parents' ability to adjust and adapt resiliently in the postnatal period. Midwives may well have limited time in which to have an impact, and this is exactly why it is so important to ensure that communication skills are prioritised.

The postnatal period is not always afforded the respect it is owed, having in the past been called the Cinderella of the service and not without good reason. Recent guidelines have tried to address issues such as women not having adequate basics including food, drink and pain relief (NICE, 2021). This is not surprising when the current reality in the UK is that women and birthing people are transferred to the postnatal wards quickly following birth. Postnatal wards are often understaffed due to the need to prioritise staffing levels on the labour ward where there is a requirement for one-to-one care. It can feel jarring for women to come from the intense support on offer on the labour ward to a postnatal ward where one midwife may be caring for the whole ward. The Royal College of Midwives (RCM) acknowledged that investment in postnatal services was necessary; however, the chronic shortage of midwives in the UK means that this will continue to be an area of struggle, along with the rest of midwifery services. The shortages have continued despite the workforce trying to make their voice heard through social media, petitions and even demonstrations. Now the MBRRACE-UK (Mothers and Babies: Reducing Risk Through Audits and Confidential Enquiries Across the UK) data have exposed the fact that women are more likely to die in the postnatal period than any other time in childbearing. Additionally, mental health is of particular concern, with death by suicide being the highest cause of maternal death in the year following childbirth (Knight et al., 2020).

It is, however, notoriously difficult to adequately prepare parents for the reality of postnatal life. A huge amount of money and time is invested by parents-to-be in preparing for the life event of starting a family. Birth preparation classes provide an excellent opportunity for building a support network and learning about labour and birth. Most private courses will include infant feeding and the fourth trimester, and while a couple of hours dedicated to the subject is better than nothing, for it to be effective, it needs to be in the context of an ongoing conversation with their midwives.

### COFFEE BREAK ACTIVITY

- What does your Trust offer to women and birthing people in terms of postnatal preparation?
- What other options are there in your area and what might be some of the barriers experienced in accessing them?

The reality is that a majority of parents do not access antenatal classes at all. In 2019 only a third of women attended NHS antenatal classes when offered, a further third were not offered classes at all and the remaining 40% were offered but did not attend, the reasons for which were not explored in the data (Care Quality Commission (CQC), 2020). There is currently no obligation on NHS Trusts to provide antenatal classes and so this results in huge differences in provision across the UK. Parents attending private classes account for an even smaller number and so the overall antenatal education landscape in the UK is generally sparse.

Consequently, parents have to rely on other sources such as social media, which means the minimal opportunities parents get to think about the postnatal period are through small, rose-tinted windows, offering no clear insight into life after birth and at worst perpetuate the idea of perfect parenting. Parents may now even experience the great American import of the 'baby shower' but even then, the reality of life with a postpartum body and a newborn baby, in a brand-new family setup, is glossed over with funny games and gender-specific gifts. Infant feeding is reduced to a binary choice between breastmilk and formula, disregarding the often agonising and complex experiences of parents trying to do the best for their babies. The topic of perinatal mental health is still shied away from despite the stark MBRRACE-UK statistics, and women and birthing people are bombarded through social media with pictures of impossibly slender postbirth bodies and contented, 'Instagram-ready' babies.

## Case Study

Ellyn gave birth to Sonny 12 days ago and the midwife is now with her for her discharge appointment. She disclosed to her midwife earlier in the pregnancy some feelings about body dysmorphia. She is feeling anxious now as she had expected her tummy to have 'gone down by now' and asks the midwife when she will be back to normal.

She wanted to try breastfeeding and it has gone ok so far; her partner has given the baby a couple of bottles of expressed milk because they want to give her a break. The baby appears well, feeds regularly, has normal yellow stools and has gained weight. Ellyn asks how she will know she has enough milk.

## QUICK REFLECTION

How might you respond to Ellyn and what will your care episode look like in this scenario?

## Body Image and Postnatal Recovery

When women and other birthing people look to the media for insight into early newborn life, they will often see 'Instagram-worthy' images of 'spring-back' bodies and 'good' babies. Even Kate Middleton, modern-day British royalty, was not able to escape the tyranny of having to appear perfect within days of birth and was paraded, much like her mother-in-law, on the steps of the Lindo Wing for the world to see. Celebrities, whether intentional or not, communicate the societal expectations that pregnant bodies, once safely delivered of their babies, must be subdued and brought back under control immediately.

## QUICK REFLECTION

Think about the last time you saw images of celebrities who are pregnant.
- What were these images communicating?
- How might you imagine a pregnant woman or birthing person might feel on seeing those images?
- Consider Ellyn's response to these images.

Popular celebrity magazines are frequently filled with images of pregnant bodies alongside observations about how to 'show off' your bump and what clothes flatter the pregnant body. These are often sat in direct juxtaposition within the same publications, where celebrities are either praised or vilified for their varying successes at casting off the 'baby weight'. In this way the media appears to both love and abhor the pregnant form and this can be a confusing space to exist within. Women and birthing people are told that pregnancy is acceptable so long as you are beautiful, but even the beautiful people need to hide away the evidence of pregnancy as soon as they can. These observations, depressing as they are, shine a light on the messages being communicated to women and birthing people throughout their maternity experience. Awareness does not necessarily equate wisdom in how to counteract these messages. However, it does allow midwives to seek to avoid a reductionist approach of dismissing the prevailing culture as irrelevant to midwifery practice.

It is also impossible to discuss postnatal body image without considering the impact of systemic misogyny which has much to answer for in the conversation about how the female and birthing body is viewed. The female form has long been objectified and seen as property to be controlled, and despite 100 years of feminism, this is still normal in everyday UK life as seen through movements such as 'Me Too'. This is mirrored in maternity where the attempt to shoehorn pregnancy and birth into linear models of control and compliance is commonplace. Women and birthing people who attempt to birth and parent outside of the accepted common medical model often face opposition from health care professionals. This despite the fact that the choices around childbearing and parenting as well as the right to choose the circumstance of birth are enshrined in human rights law (Human Rights Act, 1998) as well as in the NMC Code (2018).

In the face of such strong societal and cultural narratives, how can midwives speak positively and constructively into the postnatal period? Far from shying away from or ridiculing the role models of the time we are in, midwives need to be able to acknowledge the complexity of this period. Midwives by definition are knowledgeable about the physiology of the postnatal period. This gives them a wealth of examples of the extraordinary abilities of the birthing body to draw on. Body positivity in the postnatal period will probably look very much like drawing attention to how beautifully the body accommodates and nourishes the growing baby. Complimenting authentically and intentionally is a powerful tool of the midwife in promoting oxytocin, the hormone known to reduce stress and anxiety levels.

### PRACTICE POINTS

Think about the last time you attended a postnatal visit at a home with your midwife practice supervisor.
- How did they communicate about the physiological changes the woman or birthing person was undergoing?
- Did anything stand out to you?
- Would you do anything the same or differently?
- Did they use any phrases you found to be particularly affirming or encouraging in regard to their postnatal adjustments?
- What oxytocin-promoting comments can you think of that might encourage Ellyn to think positively about her changing body in the postnatal period?

# Postnatal Space as Transitional

Mental health in the postnatal period continues to be a complex area. After all, when you have your baby in your arms, birth trauma, bleeding nipples and often altered body image aside, women and birthing people are meant to be delighted. Birth is culturally a joyful event and parents are expected to be happy. A superficial Internet search will show you very quickly that there are a plethora of blogs and articles along the lines of 'I have my beautiful baby, so why am I so sad?' The answer is multifaceted but as with many elements of childbearing, hormones play a significant role. Oestrogen levels drop dramatically in the immediate postnatal period and combined with the transitional period of becoming a parent, this can be overwhelming. Eighty percent of women and birthing people experience what is commonly known as the baby blues (NICE, 2014) and so normalising these hormonal and emotional fluctuations is important. Discussing this in the antenatal period is ideal; early conversations highlighting the commonplace occurrence of baby blues may turn out to be immensely reassuring for those who experience it. Naming the hormones, progesterone, oxytocin and prolactin, and explaining what is happening on a physiological level may add legitimacy to the feelings of those who might feel their experience is dismissed as 'you're just hormonal'.

A potential way to help women and birthing people navigate this transitional period is to consider the postnatal period as a 'liminal' space. 'Liminality' is a term used across many professions. Architects, for example, might use it to describe hallways or airports and this illustrates the concept of being caught between two points and being on the threshold of new experiences and beliefs. The whole of the childbearing continuum is arguably a liminal space but the raw physical nature of the postnatal period catapults parents from the imagined transition to the lived experience of that transition. Navigating the physical aspects of the postnatal period can be consuming in ways women and birthing people had not experienced up to this point. This may have the potential to cause them to confront physical frailty in a way they had not considered before and this might be uncomfortable. Recovery from a straightforward vaginal birth may be faster than those having Caesarean or instrumental births, but it is a 'recovery' period all the same and needs to be acknowledged as such. Additionally, assumptions cannot be made about the rate at which a person will recover, and individualised care, possible only when women and birthing people are truly listened to, is vital.

The transition of course is not only physical and women and other birthing people are moving between two very different lives. The prebaby life may be marked by working full-time with few limitations on their time, budget and travel aspirations. For many, their main friendship network might be centred on work and so leaving this for childbearing and maternity leave may result in unexpected isolation, even more so if they don't have family living close by. In a society where stereotypical gender roles have rightly been challenged, the move from being able to set their own agenda to having the day set by a newborn and tasks becoming very domestically focused might feel disempowering. Practically speaking, the midwife can signpost to local parent and baby groups and encourage new parents to join them. Midwives cannot resolve issues of evolving identity, but they can be clear on what is and is not within their remit of support and they can listen well.

Listening is a powerful communication tool. The very act of authentic listening is a benchmark of respect. There is often limited time in postnatal appointments and using a checklist style may substantiate the belief that the postnatal period is a time to be 'resolved' as quickly as possible. This in turn may result in parents feeling like they are not being listened to or even that they are 'failing' at parenting if they or their child does not meet a standardised milestone. Listening effectively communicates respect for the person and for the process of change and enables parents to set the pace and tone, placing them in control of their own experience. It may be that due to time constraints, health professionals listen with the intention to 'answer' rather than 'hear', so active listening skills such as paraphrasing, clarifying and asking open-ended questions combined with open body language and sensitive use of silence are key to listening effectively.

**QUICK REFLECTION**

Asking open questions will result in all the answers to the physical aspect questions you need to know. Consider the different answers you might get to these questions, 'Do you have sore nipples?' as opposed to 'How do you feel breastfeeding is going?' One may elicit a one-word answer; the other is likely to tell you the full story.

What questions do you think might be helpful in helping Ellyn with her query about breastmilk supply?

## Sleeping Like a Baby

Prenatally and antenatally, parents imagine and fantasise about life with a newborn and this is an important part of bonding and forming an attachment after the birth with their child. The adjustment new parents have to make may be a letting go of assumptions they might have held about what parenting will look like for them. This may also be caught up in societal expectations of newborns.

This is not helped by questions such as 'is she a good baby?' This is often a coded question for how well the baby sleeps and how 'easy' they are. It is likely to be a well-meaning question related to an observation about the amount of sleep new parents get. However, it communicates an impression which is in direct opposition to the evidence around breastfeeding and breastmilk supply. Newborn babies from day 2 to 3 need to feed 8 to 12 times in a 24-hour period, or on average every 2 to 3 hours, day and night and on occasion, more frequently than that. Night feeds are an essential aspect of milk production due to the hormone responsible for continued milk production, prolactin. This hormone is at its highest levels overnight, making those night feeds vitally important for the ongoing supply. Therefore relating the 'goodness' of a baby to whether they sleep all night is not helpful or physiologically correct. Women and birthing people need to be provided with a realistic vision of what newborn feeding and sleeping patterns are likely to be in a way that is not overwhelming or patronising so that they can be prepared as best they can.

This question may also inadvertently cause new parents to question whether they are 'good' parents. If they are not ensuring their baby meets the imaginary standard of what being 'good' is, then they are at fault as parents. The desire to be a good parent is certainly not an unworthy goal; however, the bar for good parenting is often set impossibly high. This is particularly true when it is viewed through the lens of social media platforms and magazines and then exacerbated by continual enquiries into the 'goodness' of the baby. Additionally, various parenting theories are based on training babies into 'good' routines, so they sleep and eat on a schedule, thereby promoting a calm and enjoyable parenting experience. Again, this is in contrast to the evidence about healthy responsive feeding patterns of newborns. The message that this communicates is that if parents are finding elements of newborn life hard then they must be doing it 'wrong'. This is where the notion of the 'good' baby becomes even more problematic, because if a new parent is feeling that they are unable to describe their experience as 'good' then does that mean that they have a 'bad' baby or that they are 'bad' parents?

Midwives can be careful in their language around this and in their reactions to parents' enquiries about newborn behaviours. This again links back to making verbal associations between the physiological evidence and the present reality. Remarking on the importance of frequent feeding and night feeds at the same time as acknowledging the tiring reality is helpful. Offering careful suggestions may be even more helpful. For example, if you are asked about frequent night feeds: 'Your baby knows exactly what they are doing by feeding a lot in the night, they get to enjoy time with you as well as stimulating milk supply for the following days. It is pretty tiring though isn't it, have you tried laid down breastfeeding yet? Can I show you how?' This may then open up opportunities to talk about safe sleeping and signpost them to resources such as The Lullaby Trust. Babies who are not breastfed will still wake frequently in the night to be fed, so being familiar with the physiology and behaviours of babies regardless of feeding method is vital.

## Infant Feeding

The subject of infant feeding can feel like a perilous topic for midwives to navigate. Midwives first need to understand exactly why it is so complicated before they can truly bring a nonjudgemental approach to their infant feeding support. On one hand is the knowledge that breastmilk is the physiological norm and the best possible nutrition for babies. Breastfeeding improves both infant and maternal health outcomes globally and even a moderate increase to breastfeeding in the UK would lead to estimated financial savings to the NHS of £50 m yearly as well as thousands less hospital admissions. On the other hand is the knowledge that the current infrastructure and lack of adequate support mean that regardless of intent, women and birthing people do not get the support they need and ultimately experience the pain and trauma of unfulfilled breastfeeding journeys. Promoting breastfeeding without providing the support necessary is unfair and places the burden of responsibility with the individual when in fact as a public health issue, collective responsibility must be shared by policy makers, local authorities and NHS Trusts as well as the families. The outcome of this tension is that 8 out of 10 women in the UK are saying that they stopped breastfeeding before they wanted to and that the reasons they did so were lack of information and lack of support (McAndrew et al., 2012).

What is interesting of course is that long before these postnatal choices are being made, women and birthing people have already been influenced one way or another about breastfeeding. Influence starts as early as whether the woman or birthing person's own mother breastfed them. If they did, then breastfeeding this infant is more likely to happen (Ekstrom et al., 2003). There are of course those who benefit from the message that the way a baby is fed does not matter. Infant formula milk companies rely on the narrative that it doesn't matter how your baby is fed, as long as they are fed, and advertising campaigns focus on insecurities relating to breastfeeding such as concerns about supply and the unrealistic expectation that babies will sleep for long periods. Infant milk advertising is regulated; however, it is not uncommon for companies to make unsubstantiated claims about their powdered milks or attempt to influence health professionals through targeted advertising in health journals. Advertising is one of the most powerful forms of communication and one considered worth investing in, with over £16 m spent in 2020 advertising follow-on milks across the industry.

There are other barriers to breastfeeding and in the western world, breasts are predominantly objectified as sexual parts of the female body. Breastfeeding in public is now protected under the Kingdom Equality Act (2010); however, this has not stopped stories abounding about women being asked to cover up while breastfeeding or to move on because they are making others feel uncomfortable. Seeing as society has little issue in seeing the female form with minimal covering such as bikinis and low-cut tops, it seems likely that it is not to do with the amount of skin on show and more to do with what is being 'done' with the breasts. It is perhaps a lot to ask of the midwife to address and resolve these deep-seated societal norms; however, having an awareness of their potential influence is critical.

## QUICK REFLECTION

Ellyn has disclosed feelings of body dysmorphia. How will having an understanding of societal influences help you in your care of Ellyn?

Partners are the primary source of support for a majority of women and birthing people and so midwives ignore their influence to the detriment of the breastfeeding pair. Partners are influential both positively and negatively, ranging from fear of being excluded, feelings of possessiveness over their partner's breasts and fears of adequate nutrition (Sihota et al., 2019). While there is clearly more work to be done in terms of the objectification of female bodies, enabling partners to feel included and providing information to allay fears about inadequate milk intake are an achievable goal. Studies have found that where fathers are educated about breastfeeding and taught basic breastfeeding support skills, breastfeeding outcomes are improved for the women (Maycock et al., 2013). There is limited research at present about the influence of same-sex (female) partners other than they are generally highly motivated to self-educate and be supportive with regards to breastfeeding (Juntereal & Spatz, 2020) and it will be interesting to see how research develops in this area over the coming years.

Including partners in the conversation about infant feeding will start to break down expectations that breastfeeding is exclusively mothers' work. The act of breastfeeding is inarguably physically down to one person; however, midwives can positively affirm the partner's role and help them to see that there are ways to support their breastfeeding partner without feeding the baby with a bottle. Historically this has boiled down to a division of tasks such as breastfeeding versus changing the nappies, and this might be seen as compensatory and patronising. Caring for the breastfeeding mother by providing food, drink and other comforts can be reframed as indirectly feeding the baby as well as taking the opportunity to sit with the breastfeeding pair. These complementary acts help those breastfeeding to feel supported and those supporting to feel more involved and useful. Suggesting activities such as skin-to-skin and baby massage may also aid in promoting relationship building between the baby and the nonbreastfeeding parent. Midwives, when asked by partners what they can do to help, can explain the physiological processes of breastmilk supply and ask them what they think they could do to support that breastmilk production. Ideally these conversations would be had antenatally and parents-to-be can discuss their expectations of support from one another in advance. Doing so may allow them to identify gaps in their support network or knowledge in advance. Teaching antenatal classes to both parents is an invaluable springboard for a positive postnatal and breastfeeding experience and any chance to be able to communicate into this unique golden teaching opportunity should be taken.

There is a risk that when we view infant feeding through a simple lens of nutrition and health outcomes, we overlook the fact that breastfeeding is not just about babies being fed. Dr Amy Brown's (2019) important work on breastfeeding grief and trauma highlighted the fact that many women will approach breastfeeding with hopes and dreams about what it means to them as mothers, for their bodies and their connectedness with their babies. To reduce infant feeding to a means of nutrient transmission dismisses the lived experience of most women and birthing people who, as seen earlier, want to breastfeed. This does mean that as midwives we need to be mindful about the way we ask about feeding intention. A reductionist question will have us asking 'How are you going to feed your baby?' which on the surface appears to be a nonjudgemental approach. However, it does not allow for the complex processes leading up to these decisions and is in fact a closed, one-word answer question. The question 'How are you feeling about feeding?' opens the door for exploration on the woman's part and enables the midwife to listen and subsequently be able to provide information and support which is meaningful. Carol Rogers, an influential humanist psychologist, believed that an essential foundation of the therapeutic relationship was the concept of unconditional positive regard. This means accepting and supporting people just as they are and, in this environment, people feel accepted and are better able to experience personal growth. Support in this environment does not mean making things 'easy' and trivialising the choices around infant feeding infantilises people and takes away the opportunity for truly informed choice. It means acknowledging that this is a complex subject, that listening well and supporting them effectively in their infant feeding journey are vital.

## Birth Trauma

Birth stories become a part of women and birthing people's fabric of life and historically this would have been as much a source of knowledge as it was a common story that connects communities. Telling the birth story allows women and birthing people to reflect on the experience and make sense of it. Sometimes pieces of that story are missing, and midwives may be able to fill in the gaps, even more so if they were present at the birth, but by providing space in which they can tell their stories and ask questions, women can put together the pieces themselves.

Unfortunately, not all birth experiences are positive and it has been found that nearly half of new mothers describe their birth experience as traumatic (Long et al., 2022). When women and birthing people go on to suffer with symptoms of posttraumatic stress disorder (PTSD) because of their birthing experience, it is commonly referred to as birth trauma. Women and birthing people will experience symptoms such as vivid flashbacks, hypervigilance, avoidance and disruptions to mood such as guilt (NICE, 2018). Traumatic birth experiences are not limited to physical damage suffered in childbearing and emergency birth and the experience of birth trauma is complex and deeply personal. Risk factors such as previous abuse, feelings of loss of control, impersonal treatment by staff and not being listened to are known to contribute. These represent preventable ways directly linked to communication skills that midwives can directly impact on the likelihood of birth trauma (Birth Trauma Association, 2021).

A significant challenge to providing care to sufferers of birth trauma is that a majority of women and birthing people experiencing this level of psychological distress are unlikely to disclose until they are at breaking point. This is related to fear of judgement from others, including loved ones and health professionals, as well as new mothers and parents experiencing difficulty in determining a reference point for 'normal' for their feelings about their experience (Slade et al., 2021).

Midwives are likely to be among the first to hear women and birthing people's birth stories and this is both a privilege and a challenge. Providing an opportunity to talk about their birth experience may act as a useful screening tool for onward referral where needed, but this must be sensitively handled to avoid it becoming another part of the tick-box approach. Active listening skills yet again come into play and must be seen as the first tool of choice in the midwife's toolkit for communication with women and birthing people. The high level of women and birthing people experiencing birth trauma means there is no room for applying blanket positivity when asking about birth stories. This means asking open questions, being prepared to listen and not try to make excuses for failures in care or get defensive if colleagues are mentioned. Avoiding terms such as 'the main thing is that you are both healthy' is vital in avoiding reinforcing the prevailing narrative that everything has to be perfect and revealing perceived weakness makes you a less able parent. For some, time is a great healer, but for others, expert help will be needed to enable them to process what has happened. For this reason, midwives must refer to specialists where able, but crucially must not compound any trauma by disempowering women and birthing people in their care through not listening or communicating in a way that dismisses their experience.

**COFFEE BREAK ACTIVITY**

Considering Ellyn's dysmorphia, think about the different ways this might have impacted on her birth experience and how you might approach discussing this now in the postnatal period.

The postnatal period can no more be reduced to involution of the uterus, baby blues and breastfeeding any more than 'life' can be reduced to eating, working and sleep. Environment, culture, spirituality, support networks and personal history all form the framework on which women and other birthing people will experience their postnatal physiology and psychology. This might be further impacted by elements such as language barriers which are another layer of care for midwives to navigate. Seeking professional interpreters rather than relying on family members is the gold standard. Holistic care, as determined by the NMC Code (2018), encompasses all of this and yet oftentimes a reductive tick-box, top-to-toe approach is taken due to time constraints and perversely, a fear of missing something.

It is true that midwives have a limited time in which to make a difference, and there are many priorities vying for attention, not least of which being the worrying statistics of maternal mortality in the postnatal period. This does in many ways increase the pressure on midwives, and the temptation to resort to tried-and-tested formulas is understandable but worth resisting in favour of individualised care. Knowing that not being listened to is a risk factor for birth trauma which can impact negatively on women and birthing people for years to come underlines the imperative for postnatal care which is built on a firm foundation of excellent communication skills.

## References

Brown, A. (2019). *Why breastfeeding grief and trauma matter*. Pinter & Martin.

Care Quality Commission (CQC). *Maternity Services Survey: 2019 Survey of women's experiences of maternity care, Statistical Release*. 2020. https://www.cqc.org.uk/sites/default/files/20200128_mat19_statisticalrelease.pdf. Accessed 24 November 2021.

Ekstrom, A., Widstrom, A. M., & Nissen, E. (2003). Breastfeeding support from partners and grandmothers: Perceptions of Swedish women. *Birth*, *30*(4), 261–266.

Juntereal, N. A., & Spatz, D. L. (2020). Breastfeeding experiences of same-sex mothers. *Birth*, *47*, 21–28. https://doi-org.ezproxy.brighton.ac.uk/10.1111/birt.12470.

Knight M., Bunch K., Tuffnell D., Patel R., Shakespeare J., Kotnis R., Kenyon S., & J. Kurinczuk (Eds.) on behalf of the MBRRACE-UK. Saving lives, improving mothers' care: Lessons learned to inform maternity care from the UK and Ireland confidential enquiries into maternal deaths and morbidity 2016–18. 2020. National Perinatal Epidemiology Unit, University of Oxford. https://www.npeu.ox.ac.uk/assets/downloads/mbrrace-uk/reports/maternal-report-2020/MBRRACE-UK_Maternal_Report_Dec_2020_v10_ONLINE_VERSION_1404.pdf

Long, T., Aggar, C., Grace, S., & Thomas, T. (2022). Trauma informed care education for midwives: An integrative review. *Midwifery*, *104*, 103197. https://doi.org/10.1016/j.midw.2021.103197. Accessed 24 November 2021.

Maycock, B., Binns, C., Dhaliwal, S., Tohotoa, J., Hauck, Y., & Burns, S. (2013). Education and support for fathers improves breastfeeding rates: A randomized controlled trial. *Journal of Human Lactation*, *29*(4), 484–490.

McAndrew, F., Thompson, J., Fellows, L., Large, A., Speed, M., & Renfrew, M. J. (2012). *Infant feeding survey 2010*. Health and Social Care Information Centre.

NICE. (2014). Antenatal and postnatal mental health. National Institute for Health and Care Excellence clinical management and service guidance CG192. Available from: https://www.nice.org.uk/guidance/cg192 Accessed 24 November 2021.

NICE. (2018). Post-traumatic stress disorder. https://www.nice.org.uk/guidance/ng116. Accessed 24 November 2021.

NICE. (2021). Postnatal care NG194. https://www.nice.org.uk/guidance/ng194/chapter/Context.

Nursing & Midwifery Council. (2018). *The code: Professional standards of practice and behaviour for nurses, midwives and nursing associates*. NMC.

Sihota, H., Oliffe, J., Kelly, M. T., & McCuaig, F. (2019). Fathers' experiences and perspectives of breastfeeding: A scoping review. *American Journal of Men's Health*, *13*(3), 1557988319851616. https://doi.org/10.1177/1557988319851616.

Slade, P., Molyneux, R., & Watt, A. (2021). A systematic review of clinical effectiveness of psychological interventions to reduce post-traumatic stress symptoms following childbirth and a meta-synthesis of facilitators and barriers to uptake of psychological care. *Journal of Affective Disorders, 281,* 678–694. https://doi.org/10.1016/j.jad.2020.11.092.

United Kingdom: Human Rights Act 1998 [United Kingdom of Great Britain and Northern Ireland], 9 November 1998. https://www.legislation.gov.uk/ukpga/1998/42/contents. Accessed 24 November 2021.

United Kingdom: Equality Act 2010 [United Kingdom of Great Britain and Northern Ireland], 1 October 2010. https://www.legislation.gov.uk/ukpga/2010/15/contents. Accessed 24 November 2021.

## Resources

https://www.birthtraumaassociation.org.uk/for-health-professional/research
> *The Birth Trauma Association was established in 2004 to support women who suffer from postnatal PTSD (PN PTSD), or birth trauma. They 'aim to offer advice and support to all women and their families who are finding it hard to cope with their childbirth experience. (They) are also dedicated to researching PN PTSD and developing better diagnosis and treatment for sufferers as well as establishing preventative measures'.*

https://www.positivebirthmovement.org/
> *The Positive Birth Movement was founded by birth activist Milli Hill in 2012 in order to counteract what she saw as an epidemic of negativity around modern birth. Through antenatal discussion groups, online courses and books such as 'Give Birth Like a Feminist' (2019).*

Kay, L., Downe, S., Thomson, G., & Finlayson, K. (2017). Engaging with birth stories in pregnancy: A hermeneutic phenomenological study of women's experiences across two generations. *BMC Pregnancy and Childbirth, 17*(1), 283. https://doi.org/10.1186/s12884-017-1476-4
> *This paper considers the effect of birth stories across two generations of birthing women. The commonality between the decades was found in the legitimising of the narrative that as long as you have a healthy baby, that is all that counts. In that respect, although the mode of story delivery has evolved, the overall message has stayed the same.*

PART 4

# Professional Communication and Personal Development

# CHAPTER 13

# Communicating With Others

Kate Levan ■ Tania Staras

## Introduction

One of the concepts that midwives most associate with their practice is that of autonomy. In simple terms, this means that midwives have control over their decision-making and are accountable for their actions and omissions. In practice of course, it is not this clear-cut. What we do and how we do it are constrained by where and how we work. The legal and regulatory framework, organisational factors, guidelines and our own skills and knowledge combine to place limits on the extent of midwifery autonomy. Importantly our freedom to act is tempered by the relationships we have with women and families; our decisions must be joint decisions made jointly with them. Midwives also work with a wide range of other professionals and occupations each with their own skills and expertise.

### QUICK REFLECTION

- Make a list of all the people you had contact with last time you were on shift: what professions/occupations were they?
- What kind of contact did you have? Small talk/admin discussions/clinical discussions/support or teaching/other?
- If you were communicating an issue or problem, was this easily resolved/ dealt with?

Working with others can be rewarding and empowering. Shared knowledge and expertise combined with mutual respect not only enhances our working lives but makes care safer. Working in a multidisciplinary team can be complex and requires commitment and skill from both the organisation and individual practitioners to be effective. Communication sits at the heart of professional relationships just as it does with clients. This chapter explores the principles and practice of communicating within and across the multidisciplinary team. It includes a discussion of escalation and managing 'grey areas' (when a situation is not a clear emergency), accountability and professional responsibility. It also considers record keeping and the role and challenges of handover, where the goal is always clear accurate information giving and planning. Finally, this chapter includes a section on responding to complaints, investigations and raising concerns. These are all areas which although stressful to contemplate or be involved in, whether as a student or experienced practitioner, are necessary to continuously improve care and patient safety. This chapter gives practical ideas for managing our involvement in a way that supports honest, transparent investigation and, ultimately, service improvement. Recent large-scale investigations such as those at Morecambe Bay and Shrewsbury/Telford (Kirkup, 2015; Ockenden, 2022) can be seen as opportunities for the maternity services in general and midwifery in particular in England to learn and improve. It is vital that we understand the issues and can respond to them in order to safeguard and develop our relationships with families. This chapter focuses on investigation structures in England, but the principles considered are applicable worldwide.

## Definitions and Principles

In the introduction we briefly discussed the importance of the idea of autonomy to philosophies of midwifery. Mostly it is obvious when we are working with others, whether it is families, students, obstetricians or support workers. In day-to-day practice the relationships can seem straightforward and the boundaries clear-cut. The Nursing and Midwifery Council (NMC) in the UK is very clear about the scope of practice of midwives. If we are in a room with a labouring woman and a doctor comes in for a planned review, then we are clearly working with, and communicating with, different groups. But everything we do has a link to wider practice and to others. If we are sitting alone writing up our notes, we are communicating to the next person who will read those notes, whether in a few minutes', hours' or even years' time. Our body language when we walk out of a room conveys so much about how we are feeling about a situation even if we think nobody notices—families notice everything. Even when we know perfectly well that we are communicating with others, there are particular situations which the evidence tells us can be more challenging to perfect. Handovers can be tricky because information can be unclear, information or 'soft intelligence' can be missed and we may be misunderstood. Clinical emergencies can be challenging because we have to listen, respond and act quickly. In general when speaking in an obvious emergency, there is usually agreement about what needs to be done and how. More complex for communication and negotiation are the grey areas of practice where the situation doesn't feel quite right but is not a clear emergency. Look at these two practice examples.

**Antenatal Example**

A pregnant person presents with tailing foetal growth on symphysial fundal height measurement and plotting. As the midwife, you request an urgent ultrasound to assess foetal growth and liquor volume placental sufficiency but are informed by the ultrasound department that there is no availability.
- How would you manage communication in this case?
- Where does your responsibility lie?

**Labour Care Example**

You are caring for a woman in labour. She has a raised BMI, gestational diabetes and is having an induction of labour. She is on a continuous cardiotocograph (CTG). You are concerned that the CTG has been suspicious for a while. You have asked for an obstetric review, but the labour suite is busy and nobody has yet made a face-to-face review or made a decision as to ongoing management.
- How would you manage communication in this case?
- What do you think are the key issues?

Although both examples are challenging, they are not uncommon in practice. The principles of communication in both situations are the same—be clear about *who* you are communicating with, *what* you need and *when*. In the **antenatal example** the main issue is organisational capacity versus clinical need. The primary role of the midwife is to advocate for the client and make sure that their needs are met. In terms of communication, this means making sure that all the relevant facts are communicated to the obstetric team and asking explicitly for a face-to-face obstetric review. A discussion like this might take place over the phone—before making the phone call, make a note of who you need to speak to and exactly what issues you need to raise. Try not to end the call without a clear plan being made, and document who you spoke to, what was agreed and in what time scale. Make sure that you then communicate honestly to your client. It is worth considering making the call in a different room to the client, as overhearing these types of discussions may be stressful for the client as they may feel that they are a burden or that their needs are not as great as others. The **labour care** example also requires clear and explicit communication. It is easy to tell ourselves that in a busy labour ward our problem isn't urgent and can wait. However, we need to trust our instincts and consider our professional responsibility; if a situation doesn't feel right, then it isn't right and would benefit from a wider review and discussion. In communicating our concerns, it is vital to use the correct terminology and accurately to convey our concerns and the reasons for them. In this case, don't say 'I'm a bit worried about my CTG', try 'I'd like you to come to see client X as they are high risk with a raised BMI, GDM and is an IOL. The CTG has been suspicious for the past hour as the variability is less than 5 and it is not improving, I think she may need delivering'. This is unambiguous and makes it harder for people to say 'no'. Following review, a care plan should be developed following discussion with all concerned, including the family, explaining the rationale for it and the risks and benefits of taking action or not.

The examples both highlight the key reasons for ensuring that communication between professionals is effective. The first reason is that good communication mitigates the *risk* of situations. Knowing what, when and how to escalate concerns can be challenging but is vital in preventing further harm down the line. The issue with grey areas in practice is that they are open to different ideas and expectations—one professional might be very concerned about a situation and want to intervene whereas another may be more relaxed and happier to take a wait-and-see approach. Never forget that you are the person who knows the client best, you have spent the most amount of time with them and have a holistic view of what has been happening over the past hour. Clear lines of communications, structured discussion tools and respect between professionals can prevent these differences having a detrimental clinical impact. There will be times when unnecessary intervention occurs or when it should have occurred but hasn't. The goal of effective team working and communication is to reduce to a minimum both possibilities. The second reason is that regardless of the situation or the outcome, good communication can mitigate *trauma*. Key points raised by the Ockenden report were that women and families did not feel listened to and that when difficult or distressing events occurred there was little done to communicate honestly. Not knowing or not understanding can contribute to trauma because it becomes impossible to process events. Clear communication is therefore vital, and this includes honesty even if things are not positive. It is human nature to reassure people or dismiss their worries with the best motives, but although these actions can seem kind, they have the potential to cause further distress.

Table 13.1 shows a typical chain of communication for a midwife on labour suite who is concerned about a person in their care. This process of escalation allows for fresh eyes at every stage and also ensures that the organisation of workload on labour can take account of a potential emergency situation. The labour suite coordinator and medical team are aware that there might be a need for further intervention, operative procedures or ongoing intensive support.

TABLE 13.1 ■ **Typical Escalation Plan for Deteriorating Patient or Ongoing Clinical Concerns in Midwifery.**

| Definition | First Line | Second Line | Third Line |
| --- | --- | --- | --- |
| Escalation of care is the recognition of deterioration and communication to a senior medical or midwifery colleague, resulting in an individualised management plan. | Midwife in charge of the shift, i.e., labour ward coordinator | Senior registrar on call | Consultant obstetrician on call |

# Speaking Versus Silence

As we have seen in the labour care example earlier, it can be easy to take a wait-and-see approach rather than communicating our concerns about a person in our care. We might do this for a number of reasons. There may be times when our knowledge and experience lead us to believe that the situation will remain stable or will be resolved safely. For example, in caring for a primigravida who has been in active second stage for 2 hours, we may be aware that hospital guidelines expect us to ask for a medical review with a view to expediting the birth. However, we also know that the woman and baby are both well and safe; the foetal heart is reassuring and the woman is coping well and not exhausted. We will also be aware that the clinical features suggest that birth will take place—descent of the presenting part is occurring. In this situation we may feel that a wait-and-see approach is appropriate because our knowledge, skills and experience suggest that the situation remains within normal parameters. As regards communication and decision-making, it is vital that the woman and her labour supporter are aware of our assessment and care planning and are themselves actively involved in ongoing decision-making. We also need to be aware of the need to document our assessment of the clinical picture together with a plan and review time. In considering a review time, we must be alert to the fact that the situation may develop quickly, and we need to remain open and flexible in our approach.

In this situation, it is obvious that we as the midwife take full responsibility. The situation becomes more complex when we do ask for the review of a case but the response we receive does not feel appropriate. Consider the following case.

---

**Case Study**

**Mother With MEOWS Score of 12—Sepsis Suspected—on a Busy Antenatal Ward**

One of the women you are caring for on a busy antenatal ward appears to be deteriorating with a MEOWS (Modified Early Obstetric Warning Score) score of 12. You suspect sepsis and escalate your concerns to the midwifery clinician in charge of the shift. They recommend repeat observations in half an hour. You are unhappy with this advice as workload means that you are not able to provide 1:1 care for the woman on the antenatal ward, and you feel that she needs to be moved to the labour ward. You explain this to the midwife in charge, but their decision remains the same. You calmly explain that you wish to discuss the case further with an obstetrician and bleep the on-call registrar who is currently on the labour ward. They review the situation over the phone and agree that the woman should be transferred to the labour ward for 1:1 care and a full obstetric review and multiprofessional care plan.

*Reflection on this:*
- How will you approach this plan with the midwife in charge of your shift?
- Would you want to talk it over with anyone else?
- How could you follow this up to ensure that there will be no barriers to communication in the future and that this is seen as a positive learning experience for all?

It can be hard to speak up and to challenge, particularly as a student or junior member of staff. There are some key ideas which can help in formulating your communication in a situation which may feel uncomfortable and stressful.

**PRACTICE POINTS**

Managing challenging communication with other professionals.
Think—assertive not aggressive:
- Take your time.
- Don't feel pressured to react immediately.
- Keep actively interested by asking what the other person needs. As you understand more about the situation, and have a conversation, you will come across more assertively.
- Use a good mix of open and closed questions, and really listen to what the other person is saying.
- 'Seek first to understand, then be understood'.

In the case study discussed, there may have been particular features which made it hard for the midwife in charge to respond as you hoped. Often, we can only see the situation that we are in—the people who we are caring for or the pressure that we feel we are under. It can be important to give consideration to the pressure that the midwife in charge of the shift may have been under at that time—were they able to maintain a 'helicopter view' or was their response more based on the fact that they were not able to give you their undivided time? They may have been dealing with other complex issues at the same time and would also have been aware of wider issues of staffing, skill mixture and anticipated workflows. None of this is to excuse wrong actions or omissions, but if we can try to see a situation through another's eyes, it can help in formulating approaches that are constructive. Most of us also work in busy environments with their own cultures, guidelines and norms of behaviour and response. It can be difficult to recognise these, never mind challenging them. In the previous case study, it would help to be aware of the culture of the organisation and to consider whether it was easy to transfer care from one area to another based on clinical need or whether there were barriers to transfer. Issues of culture can be very deep seated. In this situation, it could be beneficial to discuss the issue at a unit meeting to understand and remove any possible barriers to transfer. Culturally it would be most effective if all concerned were able to discuss the matter openly and freely and to share ideas about patient flow and management. In practice within the NHS, this can be challenging because hierarchies and professional barriers can complicate open communication (see Chapter 3 for a discussion of how the professional identities of midwives and doctors can have an impact on communication).

# Grey Areas

As the antenatal and labour case studies at the beginning of this chapter show us, grey areas in care can cause real problems in communication. Grey areas are circumstances where there is not a clear and immediate emergency, but elements of a situation are concerning and may deteriorate to the point where an emergency develops. Grey areas can be challenging in knowing whether to speak up or remain silent. This is partly because we don't want to be seen to overreact or to be suggesting intervention when it is not clinically warranted. It can also be because of organisational or cultural factors—it may be hard to engage with the obstetric team as a respected professional or it may be that we don't want to 'rock the boat' when a unit is already very busy or short-staffed. Regardless of these factors, we always have a professional responsibility and a duty of care for anyone in our care and are required to do the best for that person within the limits of our scope of practice. It is always better to err on the side of caution and risk an unnecessary referral rather than to sit on something and miss the point of safe and effective intervention. Routine reviews such as 'fresh eyes' whereby a peer will regularly review a cardiotocograph (CTG), for example, can be helpful in making sure that familiarity doesn't mean we miss a changing situation. These routine reviews can also help in ensuring that there is a team approach to discussion and decision-making.

---

**PRACTICE POINTS**

Grey areas which may warrant review or intervention:
- Large for dates
- Slowing of growth
- Pink liquor vs bloodstained liquor
- Suspicious CTG
- Fresh or old meconium-stained liquor
- Slow progress in first stage
- Slow progress in second stage
- Foetal tachycardia
- Borderline blood pressure
- Nonengagement with care
  And many more...

---

These practice examples point to another complication with grey areas—that they are very much in the eye of the beholder. Unlike emergencies where there will be clear obstetric drills to follow, grey areas can be dangerous because they are subjective. Generally speaking, people making decisions about whether to refer on in grey area situations are also making other decisions and juggling other elements of a workload and communication. For example, if you see someone in triage who has reported reduced foetal movements you are likely to do a CTG as the first line of management. If the CTG is reassuring, the pregnant person may then decide to go home because they have other children to collect from school. However, your unit guidelines and your professional instincts might support waiting for an obstetric review or requesting an ultrasound scan. In this situation, you need to manage competing demands to reach the most practical and effective solution. This may include taking the CTG printout and notes to the doctor rather than waiting for them to come to you or it may involve a remote review via telephone. Some units may also have centralised CTG monitoring, enabling others to view a CTG from a different clinical area. In supporting the client to go home you would clearly communicate things to look out for and when and how to contact a midwife or the hospital. Finally, you would need to be explicit in your documentation of findings, decision-making, referrals and care planning. Obstetric grey areas should not lead to grey areas in care and communication.

Time is a key factor in managing and responding to grey areas. There can be a tendency to lose track of time when caring for someone and not to be aware of the significance of time passing, even though documentation remains up to date. It is one thing to document a foetal heart reading every 15 minutes and another to be really aware of what it means and that, for example, an episode of reduced variability has in fact gone on for 2 hours. In this situation a suspicious CTG can 'suddenly' become an emergency situation with bradycardia and thick meconium draining, even though in reality the warning signs may have been present for some time. Situations like this highlight the importance of peer review such as fresh eyes, but also of the need for senior clinical oversight and a 'holistic face-to-face review', where the whole clinical picture can be assessed, rather than just focusing on one element such as the CTG (see the Healthcare Safety Investigation Branch (HSIB) Intrapartum Report for examples of this; HSIB, 2021).

## Handovers

We have explored the communication issues around escalation of problems and identifying and communicating grey areas in care. These are both situations when effective, clear communication is vital because they involve handing over information and sometimes care from one person to another. Of course, handovers happen throughout the working day, including at set times of shift change. Evidence suggests that handovers can be a challenging time for care (Spranzi & Norton, 2020). This can be due to the effect on the work of the ward—time spent on handover is time spent away from giving care. It can also be due to what and how communication takes place—important information might be missed or misunderstood. Kirkup and Ockenden both highlight communication failures around handover as contributing to challenging situations and adverse outcomes. Traditionally handover in areas such as the labour ward has primarily taken place away from the bedside, although there are increasing moves to meaningful bedside handovers which involve families in information giving and sharing. There have also been moves towards multidisciplinary handovers on the labour ward, rather than separate handovers for midwifery and obstetric staff. However, operational issues, including different shift start times and lengths for the two groups, can make this complex and risks introducing yet more handovers and opportunities for error. Over recent years tools have been developed to assist practitioners in managing handover communication in all areas of the health service in the UK. In a review of the published literature around maternity handover, Spranzi (2014) found that the use of structured tools and mnemonics can have positive impacts on the clarity of handover and on patient safety.

---

**COFFEE BREAK ACTIVITY**

Think of your last experience of handover on the labour ward.
- Who were you handing over to?
- Did you use a handover tool?
- Did you include the family in your handover?

---

The SBAR mnemonic is one of the most widely used in obstetrics. It was originally developed for use by the US Navy and taken up by the NHS (NHS England, 2018). Table 13.2 defines what SBAR is and when the NHS recommends it should be used.

The following case study demonstrates how SBAR can be used in a practice situation.

---

TABLE 13.2 ■ The SBAR Tool for Communication.

The SBAR tool for communication:
- Situation
- Background
- Assessment
- Recommendation

Recommended uses and settings for SBAR:
- Urgent or nonurgent communications
- Verbal or written exchanges
- Emails
- Escalation and handover
- Clinical or managerial environments

---

**Case Study**

Alex (G2 P1) aged 32 comes to triage at 37/40 weeks' gestation with a history of abdominal pain and fresh vaginal bleeding.
- What observations would you take?
- What information would you gather from Alex?
- What key things would you consider in communicating with members of the multidisciplinary team in this case?

---

Think about how you would use SBAR in this case study to communicate relevant information clearly. The following is an example:

- Situation—I am calling from triage, a 32-year-old P1 has just presented with abdominal pain and fresh vaginal bleeding at 37/40.
- Background—Uncomplicated pregnancy, previous normal delivery at term.
- Assessment—I think she may be having a placental abruption, the CTG is abnormal.
- Recommendation—I would like you to come to triage and review her immediately.

Remember that other professionals are not the only people you need to communicate with in this scenario. Alex and their partner also need to understand the situation and your concerns in language that is clear and honest. Look at this explanation given to Alex:

*We are concerned that there may be a problem with the placenta or blood flow to your baby, and your baby does not seem to be 100% happy at the moment. I have asked the doctor to come immediately to see you. I will stay with you until they come and if necessary, I will ask for additional help.*

There are many ways of giving information and you may choose different phrasing, but the key is that your communication leaves no room for confusion. It is important not to use medical terminology with families as they will likely not understand it, especially as they may be anxious and be struggling to take in any of what is being said. To balance this, it is also equally vital to let families know as soon as you become aware that there is a potential problem, as families have talked about being completely unaware of a problem, maybe even watching TV in the room, and the next minute the room is full of people and the woman or birthing person is being wheeled to theatre! Ultimately, families want to know the truth and the facts of a situation relayed to them calmly and quietly using language they understand and acknowledging that they will be distressed and possibly panic. Information may need relaying several times or need to be repeated in slightly different ways as it can take time to hear and process it when people are anxious and stressed. Chapter 11 in this book looks further at the use of SBAR on labour suite and Chapter 9 explores the importance of clear and honest communication with families to reduce the risk of trauma.

# Professional Support and Debriefing

When emergency situations occur and when outcomes are poor, our first duty of care and communication is clearly to the families. They need to be supported in a way which is meaningful and empathetic (Chapter 9 has more detail on how we can achieve this). However, as professionals involved in the event, we will also need the opportunity to debrief and to be supported. This can be just after the event through a **Hot debrief**. This should take place as soon as possible after an event and involve as many members of staff as possible who were involved. Staff may be shocked, upset, confused and need support. This debrief should be facilitated by the shift leader and should give people space to acknowledge their feelings and get support from peers. Further down the line, a **subsequent debrief** should take place. This may be after any investigation has concluded. This will have given people more time to reflect and any findings or recommendations from the investigation may be starting to be implemented. This debrief will allow people to come together and reflect back but also to look forward in order to learn lessons for future care.

A recent study by Buhlmann et al. (2021) has highlighted the long-term impacts that involvement in critical incidences can have on nurses and midwives. Debriefs can mitigate this, but so can social and professional support. Always remember the core principles of professional communication when seeking support—think about confidentiality, respect and honesty.

## PRACTICE POINTS

Sources of support after critical incidences:
- Peers
- Senior midwives
- Practice supervisor/coach/named support
- Family
- University tutors or support services if applicable
- Trade Union representative (be cautious as this can imply liability)

## COFFEE BREAK ACTIVITY

- What is the process of managing complaints in your workplace?

# Complaints and Investigations

Investigations into maternity care are not new. The systematic analysis of maternal deaths in order to learn lessons and improve care goes back to the 1930s and continues today (McIntosh, 2012). However, for staff and students, the thought of being involved in an investigation or complaint can be incredibly stressful. We know that our actions and omissions will be scrutinised. Traditional structures of investigation have tended to focus on the individual and have left people feeling that they are blamed for errors or untoward incidences. Obviously there are times when individual mistakes have serious implications for health and care. Generally speaking, however, problems are multifaceted and involve more than one person. For example, a drug administration error is clearly the responsibility of the person who gave the medication. However, there are likely to be wider factors that contribute to the error. These might include poor labelling or storage of drugs (for example, two different preparations which have very similar packaging); shortage of staff or poor skill mix (which might mean that a midwife gets called to an emergency in the middle of undertaking a medicines round); or ineffective or unclear prescription writing (for example, confusion between generic and brand names for a medicine). An open and honest investigation should look at systemic issues and human factors rather than just apportioning individual blame. In this way, wider lessons can be learned, and care improved.

In recent years individual complaints by families have led to wider investigations—these include the Kirkup and Ockenden Reports. There are many different types of investigations, but increasingly external investigations are favoured because they are more likely to be impartial and less likely to blame individuals than internal or profession-based routes. In 2017 the HSIB was created and is hosted through NHS England NHS Improvement (Department of Health, 2017). Since 2018 HSIB Maternity has carried out investigations nationally and to date it has completed over 1500 maternity investigations (HSIB, 2022). Table 13.3 gives information about the work of the HSIB in maternity.

Communication is key in managing your response to a complaint or being involved in an investigation. Table 13.4 gives information about how HSIB carries out investigations and what it means for you.

Regardless of who is carrying out the investigation or why it is happening, your role is always to be open and honest about the facts as they relate to your practice or organisation. This can feel scary but as organisations internationally move towards structured approaches which do not simply blame individuals then we can begin to see investigations as part of learning and improvement rather than a potential punishment.

## Accountability in Midwifery

There are times when we may feel swept along during challenging clinical incidences, complaints or investigations. However, there are other times when we may believe or know that something is wrong in relation to the practice of an individual or the structure of an organisation. In the UK, health professionals are legally bound to raise and escalate concerns; it is a central clause in the NMC Code, which says nurses and midwives must **'act without delay if you believe that there is a risk to patient safety or public protection'** (NMC, 2018, clause 16). Students as well as qualified practitioners have a duty to speak out (Milligan et al., 2017).

## TABLE 13.3 ■ The Work of the HSIB in Maternity.

'Our maternity investigation programme is part of a national action plan to make maternity care safer. We undertake approximately 1,000 independent maternity safety investigations a year to identify common themes and influence systemic change.

- We have been tasked with carrying out these maternity investigations because we are in a unique position as a national and independent investigating body to:
- Use a standardised approach to maternity investigations without attributing blame or liability.
- Work with families to make sure we understand from their perspective what has happened when an incident has occurred.
- Work with NHS staff and support local trust teams to improve maternity safety investigations.
- Bring together the findings of our reports to identify themes and influence change across the national maternity healthcare system.

All NHS trusts with maternity services in England refer incidents to our team.'

*HSIB*, Healthcare Safety Investigation Branch.
Source: HSIB. (2022). *Maternity investigations.* https://www.hsib.org.uk/what-we-do/maternity-investigations/

## TABLE 13.4 ■ HSIB Investigations—Being Interviewed.

- **Why?** Interviews are carried out to help the investigators to fully understand the details of the event/incident.
- **How?** Either face to face or more likely virtual, you will be invited to share your recollection of events and or additional insight into how your organisation works and respond to questions. Interviews usually last between 45 minutes and 1.5 hours.
- **Process:** The interview will be recorded; this is to enable the investigators to listen back to interviews whilst preparing the report. You will be sent information before the interview around how the recordings are stored and who may request access to the recording as this is governed by Information Governance and GDPR (General Data Protection Regulation) Law. You can choose to have someone with you for support as long as that person is bound by the same confidentiality agreements as clinical staff (e.g., Professional Midwifery Advocate (PMA)).
- *The purpose of the interview is not to 'trip you up' or to apportion blame or liability; it is part of a fact-finding exercise. It is always better to be completely open, honest and transparent during an interview. Your identity will not be disclosed and HSIB reports are anonymised; they do not state the names of anybody, any Trust, family or staff member. The investigations are system based and looking at learning for the trust, not for individuals.*

*HSIB*, Healthcare Safety Investigation Branch: *PMA*, Professional Midwifery Advocate.

The Nursing and Midwifery Council sets standards about when it is appropriate to raise concerns on page 17 of the Code (2018), Nursing and Midwifery Council:

**16 ACT WITHOUT DELAY IF YOU BELIEVE THAT THERE IS A RISK TO PATIENT SAFETY OR PUBLIC PROTECTION**

To achieve this, you must:

**16.1** raise and, if necessary, escalate any concerns you may have about patient or public safety, or the level of care people are receiving in your workplace or any other health and care setting and use the channels available to you in line with our guidance and your local working practices

**16.2** raise your concerns immediately if you are being asked to practise beyond your role, experience and training

**16.3** tell someone in authority at the first reasonable opportunity if you experience problems that may prevent you working within the Code or other national standards, taking prompt action to tackle the causes of concern if you can

**16.4** acknowledge and act on all concerns raised to you, investigating, escalating or dealing with those concerns where it is appropriate for you to do so

**16.5** not obstruct, intimidate, victimise or in any way hinder a colleague, member of staff, person you care for or member of the public who wants to raise a concern

**16.6** protect anyone you have management responsibility for from any harm, detriment, victimisation or unwarranted treatment after a concern is raised NMC (2018)

Under UK law, whistle-blowers can be legally protected if they are raising concerns about their workplace (see *Raising concerns: Guidance for nurses, midwives and nursing associates* - The Nursing and Midwifery Council (nmc.org.uk), for more information about the criteria and process). Speaking out can feel very challenging. It can be worth practicing raising theoretical issues with peers to explore how you might go about talking about emotive situations in a nonemotive and professional manner. Ultimately, however, having the courage to speak out is more important than the detail of how we speak.

## Conclusion

This chapter has explored communicating with others. It has focussed on interaction with the multidisciplinary team, and has considered escalation, grey areas and handover as particular issues. Case studies and practice points help practitioners to explore and develop their knowledge and skills. This is vital because recent reports into the English maternity services have highlighted poor communication between professionals as significant areas of risk. The chapter has also explored the principles and practice of investigations and raising concerns in the maternity services. As always, open, honest communication is at the heart of everything we do—it is both challenging and vital in stressful or complex situations when something has gone wrong or outcomes have been poor. This chapter has offered practical ideas for managing our involvement in a way that supports honest communication and investigation and, ultimately, the care and safety of people and families.

## References

Buhlmann, M., Ewens, B., & Rashidi, A. (2021). The impact of critical incidents on nurses and midwives: A systematic review. *Journal of Clinical Nursing, 30,* 1195–1205.

Department of Health. *Safer maternity care: The National Maternity Safety Strategy – Progress and next steps.* 2017. https://assets.publishing.service.gov.uk/government/uploads/system/uploads/attachment_data/file/662969/Safer_maternity_care_-_progress_and_next_steps.pdf

Kirkup B. *Morecombe Bay investigation report.* 2015. https://www.gov.uk/government/publications/morecambe-bay-investigation-report

HSIB. (2021). National Learning Report: Intrapartum stillbirth: Learning from maternity safety investigations that occurred during the COVID-19 pandemic, 1 April to 30 June 2020. https://www.hsib.org.uk/investigations-and-reports/intrapartum-stillbirth-during-covid-19/?msclkid=356335afcea811ec9d4d00afdcce376b

HSIB. *Maternity investigations.* 2022. https://www.hsib.org.uk/what-we-do/maternity-investigations/

Milligan, F., Wareing, M., Preston-Shoot, M., Pappas, Y., Randhawa, G., & Bhandol, J. (2017). Supporting nursing, midwifery and allied health professional students to raise concerns with the quality of care: A review of the research literature. *Nurse Education Today, 57,* 29–39.

McIntosh, T. (2012). *A social history of maternity care.* Routledge.

NMC. *The code.* 2018. https://www.nmc.org.uk/standards/code/

NMC. *Raising concerns: Guidance for nurses, midwives and nursing associates.* 2021. https://www.nmc.org.uk/standards/guidance/raising-concerns-guidance-for-nurses-and-midwives/

Ockenden, D. (2022). Ockenden report – Final: Findings, conclusions and essential actions from the independent review of maternity services at The Shrewsbury and Telford Hospital NHS Trust. Her Majesty's Stationery Office (HMSO). https://assets.publishing.service.gov.uk/government/uploads/system/uploads/attachment_data/file/1064302/Final-OckendenReport-web-accessible.pdf. Accessed 12 April 2022.

Spranzi, F. (2014). Clinical handover on labour ward: A narrative synthesis of the literature. *British Journal of Midwifery, 22*(10), 738–745.

Spranzi, F., & Norton, C. (2020). From handover to takeover: Should we consider a new conceptual model of communication. *British Journal of Midwifery, 28*(3), 156–165. https://doi.org/10.12968/bjom.2020.28.3.156.

## Resources

HSIB Maternity programme year in review 2020/21: Summary of highlights, themes and future work 2021. https://hsib-kqcco125-media.s3.amazonaws.com/assets/documents/HSIB_Maternity_programme_year_in_review_2020-21_Report_V29.pdf
   *This report gives information about how HSIB maternity operates and the main findings from its investigations in 2020/2021.*

NHS England. *Safer care – SBAR – Situation, background, assessment, recommendation – Implementation and training guide.* 2018. https://www.england.nhs.uk/improvement-hub/publication/safer-care-sbar-situation-background-assessment-recommendation-implementation-and-training-guide/

*This guide explores what SBAR is and how it can be used in structuring clinical communication across the NHS. Although there has been some criticism of SBAR as a tool in maternity (see Spranzi, 2020, in the reference list for this chapter) it remains one of the most well-known and widely used tools.*

# CHAPTER 14

# Spreading the Word

Tania Staras

## Introduction

Earlier chapters in this book have explored the theoretical basis of communication in midwifery and its practical application to different groups of people and in different situations. Midwives and other caregivers do not work in isolation, and chapters have included discussion around communicating with the multidisciplinary team and with other agencies. This chapter extends the focus even further and explores how we can communicate with audiences beyond the bedside. Midwives are uniquely placed to tell stories of care, of birth and of their profession. We can do this by engaging in academic research and speaking and writing about that. But we can also spread the word much more widely. This chapter considers who our different audiences might be and examines communication principles and strategies for reaching out to groups and individuals, including students, the general public and academic or practice audiences. Additionally, we take a critical look at social media and the opportunities and challenges of using this to talk about midwifery in a way which integrates our professional standards and regulations. Finally, there is a section exploring communication through presentations, posters and writing for publication. Writing, speaking and teaching about what we do can sometimes seem like a chore, but it can be creative, incredibly satisfying, fun and important. Sharing the word about midwifery, however you do it, can give you lightbulb moments, changing your thinking and your practice. Getting published, supporting a student or giving a talk can extend the life and reach of your ideas—offering a spark to other midwives, women and researchers. We all have wisdom to share and stories to tell. Sometimes the smallest ideas can have the greatest impact and this chapter will help you to think about how to spread the word.

### COFFEE BREAK ACTIVITY

You come across a new issue or situation when you are in practice.
- Where do you go first for information about it?
- How do you develop your understanding and knowledge about the issue?

## Communicating Beyond the Bedside

Regardless of who we are communicating with, if we are doing it in a professional capacity then there are key principles to remember no matter what form the communication takes. The simplest approach is to make sure that we are always upholding the requirements of whatever professional regulation we work under—for midwives in the UK, this will be the *Nursing and Midwifery Council (NMC) Code*. Later in this chapter, we will look at the attributes of the *Code* in relation to the specific issue of communicating through social media. In general, however, the *Code* gives us a lot of key points to bear in mind when communicating. Of course, it may not apply to all readers, who may fall under other regulations or none, but the point of the *Code* is that it sets out broad ethical principles which have wide applicability.

The *NMC Code* has a subsection which talks specifically about communication for nurses, midwives and nursing associates (NMC, 2018):

### 7 Communicate clearly

To achieve this, you must:

**7.1** *use terms that people in your care, colleagues and the public can understand*

**7.2** *take reasonable steps to meet people's language and communication needs, providing, wherever possible, assistance to those who need help to communicate their own or other people's needs*

**7.3** *use a range of verbal and non-verbal communication methods, and consider cultural sensitivities, to better understand and respond to people's personal and health needs*

**7.4** *check people's understanding from time to time to keep misunderstanding or mistakes to a minimum*

**7.5** *be able to communicate clearly and effectively in English*

This is ok as far as it goes—it is easy to imagine how these principles can guide us in managing encounters at the bedside, in the clinic or in the home. However, further on in the *Code* is a section which gives us a much broader view of what good and effective communication should include—and what it should leave out. This final section of the *Code* is titled 'Promote Professionalism and Trust'. This is where key ethical ideas about communication are set out and which we can carry into all aspects of communications, whatever our role and wherever we work—not just those which involve clinical care. We will look briefly at some of the key ideas embodied in this part of the Code: honesty, kindness, self-awareness and role modelling.

Section 20.2 of the *Code* asks registrants to 'act with honesty and integrity at all times, treating people fairly and without discrimination, bullying or harassment'. It is not difficult to see immediately why this matters—whatever our role, it is vital that what we say and how we act are trustworthy and done with the best interests of those around us. This is true whether we are explicitly bound by the *Code* or not. The concept does not just apply to our care of women and pregnant people, however, it also applies to our dealings with colleagues and the general public either face to face or online. The same principles apply to other statements in this section of the *Code*:

**20.3** *be aware at all times of how your behaviour can affect and influence the behaviour of other people*

**20.5** *treat people in a way that does not take advantage of their vulnerability or cause them upset or distress*

**20.7** *make sure you do not express your personal beliefs (including political, religious or moral beliefs) to people in an inappropriate way*

However, although these statements seem very clear and explicit, there are always grey areas. For example, in giving honest feedback about performance to a student, we may cause them distress. There are times when it is not possible to avoid this entirely, but if we remain aware of the students' inherent vulnerability and the associated power imbalance—because they are the student and we are the qualified practitioner—then we can work to minimise distress and to make even challenging encounters hopeful. Similarly, we may have strong feelings about, for example, the place of birth. Obviously in a clinical situation we will be cautious about what we say and will use evidence and guidelines to back up our thoughts, while ensuring that the pregnant person remains at the centre of decision-making. However, it is easy to let best practice around communication slip when communicating in the classroom, with peers or on social media. The key in managing communication across all platforms and with all audiences is constantly to reflect on what and how we communicate.

Section 20.10 of the *Code* reminds us to 'use all forms of spoken, written and digital communication (including social media and networking sites) responsibly, respecting the right to privacy of others at all times'. Again, at first glance this seems really clear, but how we define 'responsibly' is very much an individual perspective; we all have different ideas about where the boundary between 'responsible' and 'irresponsible' might lie. Furthermore, there will be times when the need and expectation to be 'responsible' will potentially conflict with the requirement to be brave, candid or to challenge attitudes and practice. This also depends on where we feel our responsibility lies—is it with the profession, the service, the people we are caring for or broader society? At times these populations may align, but there may be times when thinking and communicating honestly about practice may cause us difficulties within our profession or workplace. As in so many other areas of practice, our knowledge of ourselves—of what mattes to us and of how we see ourselves—is vital in shaping our communication in a way that is honest and true to ourselves while also caring and respectful of others. Building up a meaningful community or support, but also allowing ourselves to be open to ideas and challenges, can all help us in communicating with integrity and meaning. It is not always easy though—we all believe that we automatically follow the basic principles of communications discussed across the other chapters of this book, but once we start exploring the ethical concepts surrounding communication in the real world, everything becomes more complex. We will look in more detail about how we can use reflection and self-awareness to build our practice around communication in the next chapter.

**QUICK REFLECTION**

Think of a time you told someone what your job was—perhaps in the hairdressers or during a conversation about car insurance.
- How did the person you were talking to respond—did they ask you about your job? Did they tell their own stories of pregnancy and birth?
- How did you respond to them?

Throughout this book, we have considered some of the basic principles involved in communicating as health professionals and people giving care. You will have come across these time and time again, and their application, and sometimes their complexity, has already been explored in previous chapters of this book. In terms of who we communicate with, then clearly women and pregnant people, families and other professionals are at the heart of our everyday encounters. But in fact, every time we have a conversation with someone about our job or our day, we are communicating what it means to us to be a midwife or health professional and how that shapes our views. One of the amazing things about being a midwife in particular is that in most cultures and in most countries, people have a clear sense of who a midwife is and of what they do. They may have different titles, different training, and work in different ways, but always there is the intersection with women, birthing people, families and babies. People have acted as 'midwives' in some way, shape or form for as long as humans have been giving birth. This means that when we communicate, we are communicating with people who already have their own ideas, beliefs and expectations about who a midwife is and where and how they work. It is important that we bear this in mind when we share our stories, our knowledge and our ideas—both in terms of deliberate communication through the workplace and accidental communication which takes place in our day-to-day lives.

The communication we undertake can reach far beyond the clinical area or even the people we meet as we go about our lives. Very often our communication can have a wider purpose—to learn and to educate; to build and reinforce communities of practice or support; or to challenge and to push the boundaries of our knowledge and understanding. We talk to students, housekeepers, porters and receptionists. If we are in education, we talk to lecturers, administrators, peers and practice supervisors. We read journals, watch TV programmes, scroll Twitter or

Instagram. Every encounter is communication. Some of these are clearly active—talking to a practice supervisor or reading this book to help in developing an essay. Others may feel more passive—watching *Call the Midwife* or scrolling social media. But they all build a picture of how we see ourselves which in turn influences how we communicate with others. The following sections of this chapter will look briefly why we should develop our broader communication skills and how we might go about doing this. We will focus on the student–practitioner relationship; reaching out, particularly through social media; and telling our stories. In doing so we will explore both how personal and how universal communication around reproduction can be.

## The Student–Practitioner Relationship
### PRACTICE SUPERVISION

Whether you are reading this as a registrant or a student, you will have had experience of clinical practice support—known as 'mentoring' or 'practice supervision'. Over time the specifics of how clinical teaching in practice have altered (for example, the move from mentors to supervisors within the NMC Guidelines for student support) but the principles remain the same. There is a lot of evidence around the importance of practice supervision—not just in terms of clinical learning but also for its impact on role socialisation, confidence building, pastoral support, and managing success and failure. The practice supervisor plays a vital role as gatekeeper to the profession which inevitability puts them in a position of power and authority over the student they are supporting. In 2019 the NMC rewrote its clinical learning requirements because it was felt that the traditional role of 'mentor', which combined a supportive educational and developmental role with a grading, judging and therefore potentially punitive role, puts both mentors and mentees in a difficult position (NMC, 2019a). The new structure allows practice supervisors to focus on student education and support, with overall judgements about suitability for progression or qualification sitting in the hands of a team of supervisors led by the practice assessor and supported by an academic assessor. The intention has been that this collegiate approach leaves students feeling more supported. The challenge of operating in a team approach to clinical learning is to be explicit about what good communication looks like and how issues and concerns can be shared and managed in a way that is appropriate and developmental. It is vitally important that the student does not feel that they have fallen through cracks in the system but feels heard and recognised as an individual.

Regardless of the system, country or culture of education, the supervisor–student role remains a vital one, but one which is fundamentally unequal and therefore needs all the openness, honesty and integrity that can be mustered to make the relationship and learning meaningful and effective.

## Case Study

Handover on labour suite. Two student midwives, four qualified midwives, one labour suite coordinator. One student goes straight over to a midwife.

**Midwife:** [smiling] *Hello you, how was your weekend?*
**Student:** *It was good thanks—I finished my essay so we went out on Saturday night. You?*
**Midwife:** *Well, I was working Sunday so you know...! What were you wanting today? Practice with CTGs?*
**Student:** *Yes, that would be great.*

**Coordinator to the second student:** *Who are you working with?*
**Student:** *Rob.*
**Coordinator:** *Rob's not in today ... had to change shifts ... [to the room] Does anyone want a student?*
**Midwife:** *I had a student all weekend, I need to catch my breath.*
**Coordinator to a midwife next to her:** *Nicky—can you take this student please.*
**Nicky:** *[grimaces] Ok...*

**Activity:**
- How do you think the two students feel in this scenario? Why do you think that?
- What aspects of communication are likely to have an impact on how these students feel?
- How else could the coordinator have approached the situation in the second part of the case study?
- Do you think the second student could have done anything differently?
- How does this scenario make you feel?

As this activity demonstrates, good communication between supervisor and student can hinge on the smallest conversations. If we don't feel acknowledged as a person, but are clearly seen as an issue or problem, then our confidence and our ability to learn and perform are affected. We will touch on bullying in the next chapter, but although this case study does not demonstrate clear bullying, the way we communicate with each other—both verbally and through our body language—sends out huge messages about our feelings and perceptions of the other person.

There is a significant body of work which has explored the experience of being a student midwife in health care and educational systems across the world. One of the early pieces of work (Begley, 2001) focused on how student midwives saw their role in midwifery in Ireland. The title of the paper, 'Knowing Your Place'—a quote from one of the research participants—is striking in how it lays bare the hierarchy of health care, with students often perceived as being at the bottom. Students in Begley's paper reported being ignored by staff, reprimanded in front of families and criticised constantly. Begley noted that criticism and negative comments about the service and workload further diminished students' belief and confidence. Some of the examples given seem quite breathtaking on paper:

**Student:** *I actually woke up one morning and discovered bruises on my arm where a staff nurse had grabbed me and pulled me out of the delivery room. And she said to me: 'the least you could have done was to have the caps off the Zylocaine, ready for Doctor X'. I nearly died …*

BEGLEY, 2001, P. 229

Nearly 10 years later, a paper by Hughes and Fraser (2011) also used a quote from a student research participant in the title of a paper about student midwives' experiences of mentorship in the UK. The quote—'there are guiding hands and there are controlling hands'—suggests that although not as overtly punitive as the relationships described by Begley, the way a mentor approached their role had—and has—a significant impact on the student experience and learning. The paper suggested that students felt that good mentors had certain qualities:

- Approachable
- Instils confidence
- Advocates for women
- Is evidence based and reflective

Clearly all of these attributes have direct relationships to communication—both content and style. The students involved in the research reflected on seemingly minor but actually fundamental aspects of communication that made relationships work and learning develop:

*Yeah, somebody with a sense of humour (laughter).*
*Somebody who makes you feel confident I think.*
*Yeah (all).*
*Confident in your own ability. Doesn't put you down. Never belittles you.*

HUGHES & FRASER, 2011

More recently an Australian paper has reflected on the relationship from the opposite side—what it is like to be the one doing the mentoring (Gray & Downer, 2021). The challenges explored focused primarily on work-related issues, such as time and space for the relationship to develop when clinical areas were busy and understaffed. Mentors also reflected on their lack of preparation and support for the role and the sense that it was seen by management as just part of the job rather than a significant role which required support and time. However, the paper did also consider the relationship between students and mentors, particularly around supporting students who were unprepared and the emotional labour of trying to meet the needs of students and families they were caring for.

Overall, for the relationship between mentor or practice supervisor and student to be as positive and productive as it can be, each participant needs to be seen and treated as an individual. This is not as easy as it sounds, particularly in busy and stressful work environments. As far as communication goes, openness and honesty will support us in developing relationships whether we are a student or supervisor.

## PRACTICE POINTS

Communicating with the student in practice
- Understand who the student is—stage of study, prior knowledge/ experience, hopes and fears.
- Understand the effect and impact of different personality types and learning styles.
- Establish clear boundaries to communication—beware of communicating through social media etc.
- Support and facilitate meaningful practice experiences.
- Reflect with the student on experiences and incidences.
- Listen as well as talk.
- Don't be afraid to be challenged and questioned.
- Consider the power of saying 'I don't know'—both to build a community of learning with the student and to make clear that there are things in midwifery that can't be known and that this can be a strength not a weakness.
- Role model through communication—attitudes, skills and knowledge.
- Be kind and respectful.

## MANAGING COMPLEXITY IN RELATIONSHIPS

There will be times when the student–supervisor relationship works productively and effectively—there is a give and take of ideas and it is clear that learning, understanding and practice are developing appropriately. However, there are other times when the relationship becomes complex, either due to internal or external factors.

## QUICK REFLECTION

### Reflection on challenging student/supervisor relationships

*Supervisor:*
- Lack of confidence in your own practice—perhaps due to newly qualified status, undermining/bullying by others/difficult or critical incident
- Clash of personality/learning style with student
- Constant placement of students, making it hard to re-centre your own practice

*Student:*
- Not adequately prepared for practice
- Over or under confident
- Struggling to development knowledge/skills/attitudes appropriate for course stage

*Both or either:*
- Challenging personal issues/circumstances
- Overstepping boundaries of professional roles—e.g. becoming friends

**Activity:**
- Either as a student or registrant, have you ever experienced any of these issues?
- What happened?
- What impact did they have on your practice experience?
- How were they resolved?

When we think about difficult conversations between students and supervisors, we often think first of the student who is not achieving in practice, the need to fail them and sometimes 'the failure to fail'. As a participant in a recent paper by Bradshaw et al. (2019) commented, relationships are personal and this can make failing a struggling student an emotional experience: 'You know there will be tears. One of the most stressful things I have ever had to endure in my whole career. I found it absolutely awful. The student she was lovely but she did not have the knowledge and the skills, no matter what I did' (Bradshaw et al., 2019, p. 32). Ultimately, failing may be in the best interests of the student at that point, and potentially of pregnant people and babies. But just as in clinical practice, effective honest communication throughout the relationship can make difficult conversations easier, as can seeking to build a community of support in practice supervision and with educators.

# Reaching Out
## EMOTION WORK AND COMMUNITIES OF PRACTITIONERS

Being a midwife in contemporary practice is a mix of working autonomously and as a team. In some areas we might feel more autonomous in our day-to-day role—being a community midwife, for example. By contrast, working with a high-dependency focus, we might feel much more strongly connected to the people around us and have more of a consensus approach to decision-making and action. Between these two points, on the labour suite midwives walk the sometimes uncomfortable line between being autonomous and responsible and following a team approach through guidelines and protocols. We can never give ourselves entirely over to what is happening in our assigned room and the care we are giving; we are always aware of the ecosystem around us: is the unit short-staffed, are all the rooms full, is there an emergency taking place elsewhere? Wherever we work, we will have moments of feeling that our communication with women and families is the central plank of our day, and others where we feel that the people we work with are our main focus even though we are trying to focus on giving care. This is inevitable in big complex systems such as the NHS, but it can leave us feeling destabilised because we have to be constantly alert and flexible; we can never settle into a particular way of working because the landscape around changes constantly. Students see this sometimes in the starkest terms—trying to communicate effectively with the midwife they are working with today, trying to do things the 'right way' as that midwife sees it.

There are communication challenges in all midwifery practice, but beyond managing conversations and encounters in practice, there is the *emotion work* we do around communicating. The concept of emotion work or labour has been used a lot in health care research to describe the way professionals use not just their clinical skills, but soft skills such as kindness, caring and empathy to manage care. As Hunter (2001, 2004) found in relation to midwifery, this hidden work is vital but can be exhausting. Communication binds together most aspects of emotion work—we use it to build trusting relationships with families quickly and effectively, to manage difficult situations, to advocate for women to our colleagues. Sometimes the act of emotion work can be invigorating and empowering, but there are times when it can leave us drained and exhausted. This can be particularly true when we are forced into positions which go against our philosophies of care and practice. For example, a midwife with a deep belief in the strength and power of people to labour and birth vaginally might feel very challenged by working in a culture that is risk focused. In these situations, as Hunter found, midwives will often take refuge in action through clinical acts rather than trying to confront the uncomfortableness of the situation. This in turn can lead to burnout because what we feel and what we do clash, causing us stress, tension and exhaustion.

One way to combat isolation in practice is to build communities of support. These can be virtual or through face-to-face support and contact. The idea of midwives supporting each other, particularly in a medically organised system, can be seen in the mid-1970s with the founding of the Association of Radical Midwives (ARM) in the UK. ARM was set up by a group of student midwives who were concerned about a maternity care system which seemed increasingly medicalised and uncaring. As one of their earliest members commented, ARM was a place of support for midwives who felt, as she described it, like 'refugees from the system' (McIntosh, 2012, p. 223).

ARM was an archetypal community of practice—a safe place for support and comfort, developing and challenging ideas and practices. In the 21st century face-to-face support still exists, but for many, online support and discussion groups can be vital, nurturing collaborative communication and practice. This might include closed groups on Facebook, for example, which are based around a particular geographical area or type of practice, but increasingly it is possible to find strength and affirmation through looser groups on Twitter or Instagram. Discussions ebb and flow, but they can be a great way to explore ideas; challenge yourself and reach out. They are not bound by location, time zone or background, which allows for broader learning and understanding across culture and communities. In the next section we will consider some of the principles to consider when communicating as a professional on social media.

## COMMUNICATING THROUGH SOCIAL MEDIA

### COFFEE BREAK ACTIVITY

- Do you use social media?
- What sites do you use?
- How do you use them?
- If you don't use social media, why is this?

Most people are accustomed to using social media in one form or another in their social lives and we are alert to the possibilities and risks of viewing or creating the perfect curated life online which may bear no resemblance to reality. Other chapters in this book have touched on the impact that images of perfect motherhood can have on people who are struggling with their identity or experience, and the same issues can have an impact on professionals. Social media is just a tool. It has many positive aspects in terms of building communities and exchanging ideas but carries its own risks and difficulties, which has made many practitioners anxious about using it professionally (Power, 2014). In the UK the NMC have suggested the range of ways in which social media can be used to support professional practice in positive ways (NMC, 2019b):

- Building and maintaining professional relationships
- Establishing or accessing nursing and midwifery support networks and being able to discuss specific issues, interests, research and clinical experiences with other health care professionals globally
- Being able to access resources for continuing professional development (CPD)

The NMC have also compiled specific guidance related to social media use (NMC, 2019b) which aligns with their broader principles around ethical practice both in relation to the public and to the reputation of the profession. It seems obvious that in order to benefit from engaging with social media, we need to be aware of our professional responsibilities when using it to communicate. In practice, however, there are always grey areas. For example, there may be forms or styles of communication which are seen as acceptable in a closed group which might cause offence or distress if posted openly.

**PRACTICE POINTS**

- Treat others online as you would in real life, with courtesy and respect.
- Consider the kind of information you are sharing and what platforms you are sharing it on. Is it an open or closed group? It is accessible to members of the public?
- Be aware of confidentiality and the rights of others to privacy.
- Remember the importance of sharing evidence-based information.
- Be open to other ideas and other points of view.
- Consider other people's perspectives—you might find something funny or uncontroversial, but others may be offended or upset.
- Avoid words and actions that could be seen as shaming, bullying or othering.
- Bear in mind that material shared online has a long life—it can be seen and shared years afterwards, even if you have changed your mind on that topic.

*Think before you post*

These are good principles to follow, but there are other powerful paths down which social media can lead us. Positive support in an online community may lead to *groupthink* and can actually make us less open to other ideas, experiences and points of view. The concept of groupthink was first identified in the early 1970s (Janis, 1972) and was defined as a mode of thinking within a group whereby certain ideas are sacrosanct and the urge to maintain group cohesion and identity comes at the cost of critical thinking. We have seen elsewhere in this book how beliefs around 'normal' childbirth may have contributed to the actions and omissions of midwives in Morecombe Bay, as highlighted in the Kirkup report (Kirkup, 2015). Groupthink means that it can be very hard to challenge the beliefs of the group, and those who do not agree can feel marginalised or pushed out. Generally speaking, no one sets out to create that circumstance but it can be easy for some voices to be heard more loudly than others and to have a disproportionate influence. When using social media, we need to be careful that we continue to be respectful and open in our approach, while also building communities of support and learning.

# Telling Your Stories

So far in this chapter, we have explored the rewards and challenges of communicating with different groups of people beyond the bedside. Midwifery has always had a strong culture of storytelling for learning, support and developing professional identities. In this section, we will look at a variety of ways of sharing our stories and knowledge with students, colleagues, the childbearing community and wider society. We will consider more traditional forms of sharing through writing for publication, oral presentations and teaching (although these can of course be presented in new ways—through blogs, vlogs and podcasts, for example, as well as traditionally paper-based or face-to-face approaches). We will also briefly mention creative approaches to communicating midwifery, including art and fiction. As always, we can only touch on ideas and issues; the resources at the end of the chapter will give you further ideas for developing your voice.

## WRITING FOR PUBLICATION

It can seem strange that we do a lot of writing in order to become midwives—that most practical of careers. We write university applications, endless essays once we are studying, personal statements for our first job ... for some the thought of writing for publication can seem daunting or unnecessary.

But as we know, we are all expected to use evidence-based practice in our work. This can be huge pieces of quantitative work, systematic reviews or qualitative studies. Quite apart from all that intense academic production, case studies and personal reflection can enrich our understanding of practice and help to develop meaningful change. Nobody should be put off writing by thinking that publishing is a specialised business only accessible to certain people. It does take a bit of confidence, but you don't have to be an academic or even a qualified midwife; students, doulas, support workers, pregnant women and people—we all have things worth sharing.

---

**COFFEE BREAK ACTIVITY**

You have undertaken a research study which asked:
*What are women's lived experiences of midwifery care in the first 24 hours after birth?*
Think about how you might share your research. What audiences might be interested?
- The public
- Midwives
- Students
- Researchers
- Lecturers
- Mangers/policy makers

1. Choose two of these groups and think about which aspects of your research they might be interested in and how you could tell them about your research.
2. Think about whether they are likely to be interested in your literature review, your methodology and methods, your findings, your discussion, and your implications for practice.

---

As this activity shows, any writing we do works best when it is effectively planned and written for its audience. The same is true of where we consider publishing our work. An academic or student might read a peer-reviewed journal such as *Midwifery*, a practitioner might choose a more practice-focused publication, and members of the public might be more drawn to a piece in a consumer publication (for example, *New Perspectives* for the National Childbirth Trust). Alternatively you might decide to self-publish through a site such as WordPress which gives you more freedom in what you say and how you say it. All these platforms and audiences have overlap but it can really help your planning if you have in mind the group you really want to reach.

When you are planning your piece, bear in mind that, generally speaking, readers will be primarily interested in the findings of your work. Keep supporting material such as the rationale for your study, practice links, ethics approvals, methodologies and data collection tools brief and clear. Of course, the detail of how much you focus on different elements depends on the audience and the journal or platform, as we have discussed earlier. For detailed ideas about how to put your work together, see McIntosh (2017).

Finally, remember that anything you write needs to find its audience—people won't automatically know that you have published something. It can be tricky but selling yourself and your ideas can be key to developing your career and maybe even changing practice. Use your social media accounts to tell the world what you have done, send copies of your work or links to practitioners and managers. You never know how reading your work might change someone's thinking.

## PRESENTATIONS AND POSTERS

Writing for publication in one form or another might be the most traditional way for professions to share knowledge but it is by no means the only way. For centuries, most midwives could not read or write (in common with the rest of the population), so knowledge was shared and developed through storytelling. We can use TikTok or YouTube to continue this tradition today, as well as oral presentations at conferences, in practice or in the classroom. These might be backed up by visual aids such as pictures or posters—or the poster might stand alone containing all the information you want to share. On the wall at a conference, in a staff room or in a classroom, a poster allows audiences to explore your ideas in their own time.

Just as with writing, preparing and giving a presentation can seem daunting but it is a powerful way of getting our ideas across—and engaging with audiences. They don't need to be long or complicated or academic—just 5 minutes talking about an idea for practice can be incredibly potent.

### PRACTICE POINTS

Giving a talk or presentation.
- Think about your audience—will they already know something about the topic or will it be new to them?
- Keep your ideas simple—one or two clear ideas only.

- If using visual aids such as PowerPoint, keep them uncluttered and don't try to include too much information.
- Focus on your main points—don't get bogged down in presenting critiques of evidence, for example. Reference lists etc. can always be included in handouts or at the end of a PowerPoint.
- Practice your timings and try to use cue cards with simple phrases on to jog your memory rather than reading from a script.
- Have confidence in what you are saying—if you believe it then your audience will too.
- If having an audience makes you nervous, then focus on one trusted friendly face or look slightly over peoples' heads so you don't have to focus on anyone.
- Enjoy any questions that come your way—people aren't trying to catch you out; they are interested in what you have said.

## CREATIVE APPROACHES: FICTION, POETRY, ART, THEATRE ...

So far, we have concentrated on sharing evidence and facts through the written and spoken word. But midwifery is as much art as it is an evidenced-informed science; storytelling and sharing emotions through fiction, poetry, art and craft have real power to teach and support us. There are some things that are beyond evidence and rely on our wider senses. Social media means that we are less reliant on traditional ways of sharing ideas, and less subject to gatekeepers who decide what can or cannot be in the public domain. While working within ethical and professional frameworks, we can use online platforms to share our creative approaches to midwifery and reproduction. Just as powerfully, we can write stories and poems, draw and paint or craft in private to help us to reflect on and perhaps make sense of our experiences. Nothing is off limits—you don't have to be an 'artist' or a 'writer' to engage in creative activities. There is increasing evidence that our mental and physical wellbeing is enhanced by working creatively, whether collaboratively or for ourselves (Gillam, 2018).

### COFFEE BREAK ACTIVITY

**Blackout Poetry**
In blackout poetry you don't need to start with a blank page and think of words to fill it. Instead, you take a page of text—a book, a newspaper, a midwifery journal article, this book, and use the words of the page to build up your poem. It doesn't have to rhyme, and it doesn't have to make sense. Use a black or coloured marker pen to colour over the words you don't need.

## A Blackout Poem (From the First Paragraph of This Chapter)

~~Earlier chapters in this book have explored the theoretical basis of communication in midwifery and its practical application to different groups of people and in different situations.~~ **Midwives** ~~and other caregivers do not work in isolation and chapters have included discussion around communicating with the multi-disciplinary team and with other agencies. This chapter extends the~~ **focus** ~~even further and explores how we can communicate with audiences~~ **beyond** ~~the bedside. Midwives are uniquely placed~~ **to tell stories** ~~of care, of birth~~ **and** ~~of their profession. We can do this by engaging in academic~~ **research** ~~and speaking and writing about that. But we can also spread the word much more widely. This chapter considers who our different audiences might be and examines communication principles and strategies for reaching out to groups and individuals including students, the general public, and academic or practice audiences. Additionally,~~ **we** ~~take a critical look at social media and the opportunities and challenges of using this to~~ **talk** ~~about midwifery in a way which integrates our professional standards and regulations. Finally, there is a section~~ **exploring** ~~communication through presentations, posters and writing for publication. Writing, speaking~~ **and** ~~teaching about what we do can sometimes seem like a chore, but it can be~~ **creative,** ~~incredibly satisfying, fun and important. Sharing the word about midwifery, however you do it, can give you light bulb moments, changing your thinking and your practice. Getting published,~~ **supporting** ~~a student, or~~ **giving** ~~a talk can extend the life~~ **and** ~~reach of your ideas -~~ **offering** ~~a spark to other midwives, women and researchers. We all have~~ **wisdom** ~~to share and stories to tell. Sometimes the smallest ideas can have the greatest impact and this chapter will help you to think about how to spread the word.~~

As health professionals, we understand the requirement that we are evidence based in our practice. But the work that we do with students, with each other and with pregnant people and families goes beyond evidence. We don't have to create for others to see, but allowing ourselves to be playful in our writing, drawing, making and acting has the potential to unlock new aspects of ourselves and enhance all areas of our practice—the Resources section at the end of this chapter has suggestions to develop these ideas.

## Conclusion

This chapter has explored communication beyond clinical encounters. We have explored the different audiences with whom we communicate and how we might approach these encounters. We have considered communication between students and supervisors, communication to teach and reach out and the rewards and challenges of using social media. Finally, we have looked very briefly at how creative communication—whether for ourselves or with others—can give us the opportunity to reflect and to grow as practitioners and as individuals.

## References

Begley, C. M. (2001). "Knowing your place": Student midwives' views of relationships in midwifery in Ireland. *Midwifery, 17,* 222–233.

Bradshaw, C, Pettigrew, J., & Fitzpatrick, M. (2019). Safety first: Factors affecting preceptor midwives experiences of competency assessment failure among midwifery students. *Midwifery, 74,* 29–35.

Gillam, T. (2018). *Creativity, wellbeing and mental health practice.* Palgrave Macmillan.

Gray, M., & Downer, T. (2021). Midwives' perspectives of the challenges in mentoring students: A qualitative survey. *Collegian, 28,* 135–142.

Hughes, A. J., & Fraser, D. M. (2011). "There are guiding hands and there are controlling hands": Student midwives experience of mentorship in the UK. *Midwifery, 27,* 477–483.

Hunter, B. (2001). Emotion work in midwifery: A review of current knowledge. *Journal of Advanced Nursing, 34*(4), 436–444.

Hunter, B. (2004). Conflicting ideologies as a source of emotion work in midwifery. *Midwifery, 20,* 261–272.

Janis, I. (1972). *Groupthink* (2nd ed.). Houghton Mifflin.

Kirkup B. *Morecombe Bay investigation report.* 2015. https://www.gov.uk/government/publications/morecambe-bay-investigation-report

McIntosh, T. (2012). *A social history of maternity and childbirth: Key themes in maternity care.* Routledge.

McIntosh, T. (2017). Turning your assignment into a publication. *MIDIRS Midwifery Digest, 27,* 3.

NMC. *The code.* 2018. https://www.nmc.org.uk/standards/code/

NMC. *Standards for student supervision and assessment.* 2019a. https://www.nmc.org.uk/standards-for-education-and-training/standards-for-student-supervision-and-assessment/

NMC. *Social media guidance.* 2019b. https://www.nmc.org.uk/standards/guidance/social-media-guidance/

Power, A. (2014). What is social media? *British Journal of Midwifery, 22*(12), 896–897.

## Resources

Davies, L. (Ed.). (2007). *The art and soul of midwifery.* Churchill Livingstone Elsevier.
*This edited book has theoretical elements but is primarily practical and empowering. Different chapters focus on different creative practices, offering concrete ideas, as well as considering the impact they can have on midwives and midwifery.*

Progress Theatre: https://progresstheatre.wordpress.com/
*Progress Theatre is a group of (mostly) midwives who use drama to tell stories about midwifery and maternity. They have been operating since 1999 and have tackled a variety of complex and taboo subjects.*

Blackout poetry: https://powerpoetry.org/actions/5-tips-creating-blackout-poetry; https://austinkleon.com/category/newspaper-blackout-poems/
*These two sites offer different approaches to using blackout poetry; the first gives tips and ideas, the second is a blog run by Austin Kleon who works extensively with blackout poetry.*

Art and midwifery: https://www.all4maternity.com/caring/blog/birth-art-culture/
*This site is curated by Laura Godfrey Issacs, a midwife, artist and birth activist. It has lots of inspiring art and ideas for developing creative practice to support our work as midwives and our own wellbeing.*

# CHAPTER 15

# Reflection, Development and Challenges in Communication

Tania Staras

## Introduction

Modern midwifery practice is challenging, complex and rewarding. As the chapters of this book have demonstrated, practitioners are required to juggle myriad ideas and principles as they go about their day-to-day work. At the heart of all these is communication. This encapsulates all other care, whether at home, in the community or in the acute setting, and whether with families, other professionals or the general public. What we say and how we say it matters. Recent reports into maternity service failings have highlighted sometimes appalling clinical care, but also the lack of humanity, care and compassion that runs alongside it (Ockenden Report; Ockenden, 2022, p. 123).

Throughout this book, you as the practitioner have been part of the story. Case studies, reflections and coffee break activities have challenged you to think about your experiences, your hopes and fears and how you might develop your practice. This chapter takes those ideas further by putting your professional and personal development around communication centre stage. The first section considers you as a practitioner, exploring what kind of communicator you are and what skills of communication you might seek to develop. The second section will examine how you can use creative reflection, support and goal setting to enhance your skills. It will suggest ideas and tools to help you in setting goals for yourself and working to embed communication skills and principles in a way that is meaningful and true to you and your practice. The final section will consider briefly some of the challenges of contemporary practice, including COVID-19, the future of midwifery and virtual communication. The section will not seek to 'solve' these issues but will consider how our skills in communication can help us to navigate and mitigate them.

# You as a Practitioner
## WHAT KIND OF COMMUNICATOR ARE YOU?

Midwives and other health care practitioners all have different styles of communicating. Some of these might be influenced by social factors such as age, gender, ethnicity, culture, education and perceived or actual social status. Some of us might be more outwardly confident in communicating with a range of people, others of us might be quieter or appear more reflective. Of course, how we communicate depends on where we are, who we are with and how we are feeling. You might feel very differently chatting over coffee with colleagues who are friends than you do handing over clinical care to those same colleagues at the end of a busy shift.

---

**QUICK REFLECTION**

Remember the first time you walked onto the labour suite as a student.
• What did it feel like?
• How did you communicate with the people around you?
Think about the most recent time you walked onto the labour suite.
• What did it feel like?
• How did you communicate with the people around you?

1. Are there differences between the two experiences?
2. Why do you think this is?

---

Some of our communication is therefore clearly influenced by external factors. Researchers have suggested, however, that we each have fundamental communication styles which have an impact on how we engage with others. A lot of the work around this focuses on management and leadership styles, but the concepts have applicability to all of us. One of the most influential writers in this area was Norton, who developed a communication style inventory in the late 1970s (Norton, 1978) and proposed that there are 10 primary styles of communication, as can be seen in Table 15.1.

---

**COFFEE BREAK ACTIVITY**

• Which communication styles do you feel most reflect your professional communication?
• Which do you feel least reflect you?

---

Most people are a mixture of these different styles, but with one or two more dominant. More recent work has built on these types to suggest that they can be grouped into main areas of communication. It is fairly obvious that the *dramatic* and *animated* styles might cluster together, as might *dominant* and *contentious*.

Work by Brown et al. (2011) in Australia on how health care students see their communication styles found that the majority self-reported as *friendly*, followed by

TABLE 15.1 ■ **Norton's Communication Styles.**

| Communication Style | Characteristics |
| --- | --- |
| Dominant | Seeks to lead and control conversations |
| Dramatic | Uses devices such as exaggerating and understatement |
| Contentious | Argumentative |
| Attentive | Taking care that others feel heard |
| Animated | Uses nonverbal cues—hand gestures, nodding, etc. |
| Impression leaving | Memorable |
| Relaxed | Comfortable and not anxious |
| Open | An extraverted approachable style |
| Friendly | This can range from not being hostile through to being intimate |
| Precise | Uses accuracy and detail |

Adapted from Brown, T., Williams, B., Boyle, M., Molloy, M., McKenna, L., Palermo, C., Molloy, L., & Lewis, B. (2011). Communication styles of undergraduate health students. *Nurse Education Today*, *31*, 317–322.

*attentive* and *animated*. They were less likely to see themselves as *contentious*, *dominant* or *relaxed*. Other research has found that *friendly* and *attentive* styles work best with patients and clients in terms of their understanding and compliance, whereas the *dominant* or *contentious* styles of caregivers lead to lower understanding and compliance.

## WHAT IS EASY/WHAT IS CHALLENGING?

Health care roles such as midwifery require certain communication styles to be effective. Similarly, particular types of people are attracted to health care roles. Very often these two elements combine—as we saw earlier, health care students rate themselves as friendly and attentive in communication style, and evidence suggests that patients and families respond well to these styles. You may have noticed this in your own practice—situations where your preferred and most natural style of communication is appropriate will feel easy, enjoyable and positive. If you see yourself as an attentive communicator, then a one-to-one situation which might involve an element of counselling will suit you. You might gravitate towards specialist roles such as breastfeeding support or birth debriefing services. Even everyday midwifery roles like labour care will be enhanced by friendly and attentive styles of communication.

So far so easy perhaps. The challenges arise when we feel pushed out of our comfort zone in relation to communication and forced to take on a style with which we don't feel comfortable. If we see ourselves as friendly, attentive and animated, we might feel uncomfortable working with people who don't use our style or for whom it doesn't work in that particular context. For example, although most midwives are very keen to support women and people using hypnobirthing techniques in labour, we are also very used to verbal communication. The silence of women who go into themselves during labour can be quite uncomfortable for those around them. As midwives, we need to recognise any discomfort we feel in situations like this and reflect on how we can manage our feelings and responses in order that our quiet presence and support have a positive effect on those around us.

## COFFEE BREAK ACTIVITY

Look at Norton's communication styles in Table 15.1. Decide which style of communication is best suited to each activity here:
1. Handing over care to a more junior colleague.
2. Breaking bad news to a family.
3. Supporting a woman through the transition phase of labour.
4. Asking a senior colleague to review a cardiotocograph (CTG).
5. Advocating to the medical team for a pregnant person who has chosen to refuse a Caesarean section recommended for clinical reasons.
6. Working with a student midwife you have not met before.

- Are there some activities on this list that you know you would find more challenging and uncomfortable?
- How could you use knowledge about communication styles to help you to develop your communication in the areas that you find more difficult?

Even more challenging might be times when we need to demonstrate courage in communication, perhaps by advocating for a person in our care or by challenging poor practice. In these situations, we may need to adopt a more dominant or precise style in order to get our points across. This does not mean becoming aggressive or rude, but it may mean taking control of conversations in a way that we are not used to. If we recognise that we gravitate towards animation as a communication style, we also need to recognise that in certain clinical situations such as handover, it might be distracting and confusing and that precise organisation and language are more appropriate. Interestingly Brown et al. (2011) noted that their health care student respondents did not generally characterise themselves as *relaxed* in style. The idea of a relaxed communication style could have negative connotations—it might be seen as lacking attention to detail and being superficial. However, as Brown et al. (2011) observed, there are times when a relaxed style could be really beneficial in health care settings. It could be used to help reduce stress and tension in difficult situations—a midwife who demonstrates that they are comfortable and not anxious during the transition phase of labour can transmit that positive emotion to the labouring person and family.

We are all a mixture of different styles of communicating and it can be worth exploring our less dominant styles in order to support our communication in all situations.

# Reflection, Support and Goal Setting
## REFLECTION AND SELF-AWARENESS

Our discussion in the previous sections relies on you having a level of self-awareness about how you communicate and the willingness to reflect on what this means to your practice and how you can develop your skills. In fact, this whole book has asked you not just to read passively, but to think and to engage with scenarios, ideas and issues throughout. We grow and develop when we have the strength and courage to look at ourselves and our practice, not just to criticise, but to understand, sometimes to accept and to learn. In order to give individualised person-centred care, we need to see ourselves as individuals.

Midwifery has a history of active engagement with the process of reflection. There are many definitions and many models available to help you to structure your ideas around your experiences. Fig. 15.1 shows some of the main ones used in midwifery.

The idea behind reflection is a deceptively simple one; it gives practitioners the tools to think critically about their practice and development, thereby ensuring both autonomy of practice and lifelong learning. Both of these concepts are hallmarks of midwifery as a profession and both are far easier to write on paper than they are to achieve in practice. There are long-standing criticisms of reflection as practiced in midwifery. Kirkham (1997) argued that far from challenging our

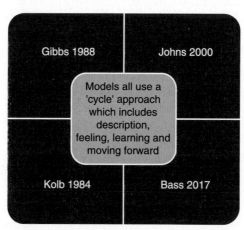

**Fig. 15.1**   See Wain (2017) and Bass et al. (2017) for more detail on how each model is structured.

thinking and developing our practice, reflection can just reinforce our preconceptions and prejudices. This is because models developed by experts lead our writing and thinking down particular channels and suggests that the process is linear, with a beginning, a middle and an end. Kirkham suggested that other forms of reflection might bring more meaningful learning—a team approach, for example, or one which actively included service users. She also drew attention to the power of creative writing and art to explore different connections and give us different ways of seeing. The use of creativity was discussed briefly in Chapter 14, together with some suggested resources.

## PRACTICE POINTS

The purpose of reflection:
- Challenges routine thinking and action
- Develops critical thinking and clinical reasoning
- Links theory and practice
  Reflection should lead to more thoughtful practice and better care for families.

Meaningful reflective practice can help us to develop our skills and understanding around communication as well as concrete clinical issues. In order to work well and be effective, reflection doesn't have to cover major events of problems. Sometimes the smallest moments can lead to the greatest understanding and to real personal change. Use the exercises throughout this book to think about the little moments and what they mean to your practice.

## QUICK REFLECTION

Next time you go into practice, take a mental note of the first few moments you have with the first client you meet—might be in community, labour ward or other clinical setting.
  You don't have to remember the conversation word for word, but try this exercise:
- What was the setting for the encounter?
- Was there anything else significant about the situation?
- What was the conversation about (might be clinical, might be the weather)?
- What do you remember about body language/nonverbal communication?
- How did you feel?
- How do you think the other person felt?
- Thinking about the principles of honesty, respect and holistic care, did this conversation achieve those?
- Do you think the other person would have felt the same?
- Is there anything you would change/do differently?

The following is an example to give you some ideas about the kinds of things we might consider and how they might help our practice around communication.

Setting: Antenatal clinic at GP surgery, very busy. Clinic running late.

Rukshana came in with her toddler in a buggy. She apologised for the fact that the buggy and her coat were very wet. I agreed that the weather was horrible and told her not to apologise. She pulled her coat off and sat down. The coat slipped on the floor and she apologised again. Again, I told her it didn't matter. The toddler in the buggy started kicking the rain cover so she unhooked it and folded it back. I said hello to the toddler who grinned at me and then hid his face.

Rukshana seemed a bit flustered. I sat at the desk and made sure that I had the right screen up on my computer.

I thought if I did this, she would feel less pressured than if I was staring at her and clearly waiting for her to sit down. I did feel anxious because the clinic was already running late. I could see the clock behind Rukshana's chair.

I wonder if Rukshana was trying to do things quickly because she knew we were running late. She clearly felt bad about coming in wet.

It was a one-minute encounter before the antenatal appointment properly started. I hoped that I put Rukshana at her ease by telling her not to apologise and by focusing on the computer rather than her. She might have felt belittled by my dismissing her apologies—as though it didn't matter, when it obviously did matter to her. Similarly, perhaps I looked impatient by tapping at my computer rather than engaging with her.

I am always aware of my language and my communication in antenatal appointments and try to make sure that people do not feel rushed—it matters that they have time and space to talk about their issues and that we can do the check-up thoroughly.

However, perhaps I need to be more aware that the tone of the encounter can be set in the first few moments.

Maybe I could move the chair so that I am not obviously glancing at the clock.

Next time I would try to show through my body language and conversation that I didn't mind—perhaps share a story of my own about the weather so she felt that I was really alongside her.

I did some reading to understand the purpose of small talk in these situations. McKenzie (2010) analysed conversations between midwives and women in an antenatal setting in Canada. Her paper suggested that 'when female health care providers attended to relational aspects of their interaction with women clients, they were able to reduce power imbalances, mitigate patient stress and improve confidence and facilitate the reciprocal self-disclosure that promotes both relational and medical goals'. I can see the value of this in terms of developing practice and will explore how I can develop my supportive conversation.

As you can see, the encounter I have reflected on is not clinically important or significant, but this tiny moment gave me a chance to consider how my words and actions might have come across and how I could develop my practice to ensure that I was respectful and holistic throughout. I could have extended this reflection by asking Rukshana for her thoughts and feelings (rather than assuming or guessing), and if I had someone else in the room (a student if I was a midwife, or a midwife if I was a student), I could ask for their feedback and ideas.

## SUPPORT

Reflection and learning don't have to take place alone. We generally work as part of a team in one way or another and as suggested in the section earlier, reflection can be even more powerful if we share it and learn from and with each other. As we have seen throughout this book, there are times when communication is uncomplicated and works, and there are other times when it can be part of much more challenging, complex or difficult situations. In these cases, it is important to remember that we can turn to others for support, debriefing and help in moving forwards. Traditionally midwives had a process of statutory supervision which worked alongside informal support structures (McIntosh, 2012). Although initially seen as wholly punitive, it was modified to try to provide holistic, supportive conversations between practitioners. The statutory model of supervision was abolished in 2015 and other processes have been developed in order to support practitioners. NHS England (2017) has developed A-EQUIP, which aims to support both midwives and families through the facilitation of different approaches to practice development (Fig. 15.2).

Professional Midwifery Advocates (PMAs) support individual midwives to reflect on and develop their practice—this includes communication in all its forms as well as clinical care.

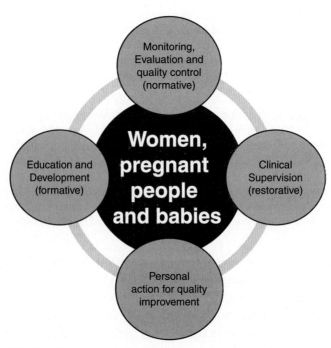

**Fig. 15.2** A-EQUIP model.

## GOAL SETTING

As we have seen throughout this book, communication is entwined with every-thing we do every day as midwives or other health professionals. We are drawn to health care practice initially because we see ourselves or know ourselves to be good communicators, with compassion, care and understanding at the heart of how we respond to the world around us. Immersion in practice builds our skills and our knowledge around communication. However, as this book has high-lighted, communication skills are often taken for granted in our work. They are not explicitly taught or discussed or reflected upon. That is not to say that they aren't part of education, training and practice, but that they are often implicit rather than explicit. This book has also highlighted the extent to which learn-ing around communication can always take place. The publication in 2022 of the Ockenden Report, together with debate about language used in maternity care, has reminded us that there are always new ways to learn and to understand. However experienced we are and however able a communicator we might be, there are always challenges and goals that we develop and strive for around our communication.

Setting practical goals can help to turn our reflection into action. Austin et al. (2020) explored how student midwives in New Zealand could be supported to com-bine reflection with goal setting reflecting on a specific incident and then using their practice assessment requirements for their level of practice to help them build meaningful goals. In the English setting, this could involve using a simple reflective cycle in conjunction with the national Midwifery Record of Ongoing Achievement and the NMC Standards of Proficiency for Midwives (NMC, 2019). There are many tools available to help with goal setting. A similar one, which you may be familiar with, is the SMART approach.

| Specific | Make sure you are clear about exactly what you want to achieve. |
|---|---|
| Measurable | Think about how you will know when you have achieved your aim. |
| Achievable | Make sure your aim can be reached. |
| Realistic | Think about what you are aiming for—not too big or too small. |
| Timeframe | Plan a realistic timeframe to achieve your goal. |

We could use this approach to set goals related to the brief reflection around the encounter with Rukshana discussed in the Reflection and Self-Awareness section of this chapter.

**SMART GOAL SETTING EXAMPLE**

**S:** Developing my skills of communication in the first few minutes of a clinical encounter.

**M:** This feels like a goal to work with clients on. I could ask for feedback from clients about how they felt about the consultation. I could ask for a peer to sit in with me and give me feedback.

**A:** Thinking about how my goal fits in the wider clinical environment.

**R:** I would like people to feel comfortable from the moment they walk into the room.

**T:** I will work on my verbal and nonverbal communication over the next two clinics and then reflect on what I have learned.

As can be seen in this example, setting goals around communication can be more complex than around, for example, developing a clinical skill such as venepuncture. This is because communication is not just about us but involves anybody we are communicating with. When planning goal setting therefore it is worth considering how you might involve families, colleagues or supervisors in developing your ideas and particularly in receiving honest, constructive feedback. Think about working with people you trust and respect—communication is so key to how we see ourselves that any criticism of our approach needs to be considered and thoughtful because it can negatively affect our view of ourselves.

**COFFEE BREAK ACTIVITY**

- What contemporary and future challenges in midwifery practice do you think need consideration?
- What impact might they have on communication in midwifery practice?

# Contemporary and Future Challenges— Responsive Communication

As we have noticed, midwifery practice is dynamic and responsive. Some of the key features of pregnancy and birth are fairly constant but medical knowledge, social conditions and care practices are in a constant state of flux. For this reason, when thinking about our practice as communicators, we need to be aware not just of our own skills and learning needs, but also of the world around us. It is important always to place our work in its widest context in order that we can be responsive and effective. This means understanding current issues but also considering how change in the near future might have an impact on how we work and how we communicate. This section of the chapter looks very briefly at some of the areas to consider when thinking about how we can develop our practice and our communication. These ideas can be fed back into reflection and personal practice development. The areas we will highlight are COVID-19, virtual communication and the future of midwifery; the list is not exhaustive and you may think of other issues which are relevant to practice.

## COVID-19

My daughter was pregnant, and gave birth, in 2020. She attended every antenatal appointment and scan alone. Her partner sat on a chair on an empty hospital corridor while she was in early labour on the ward. Hers was a normal experience for many women during COVID-19.

> **QUICK REFLECTION**
> - What do you think were the main changes to midwifery practice because of COVID-19?
> - Which changes do you think will stay part of practice in the long term?
> - How do you feel about these changes (positives and challenges)?

The pandemic has had a huge impact on every aspect of life globally, partly due to the risk and uncertainty that a new life-threatening condition has on us all and partly due to the impact of national and international restrictions on life. Many countries have experienced lockdowns of varying lengths and severity, with the opportunity to communicate face to face being severely curtailed in social, work and caring situations. In the UK, in common with many other countries, access to in-person care was significantly curtailed, visitors and birth companions were largely removed or restricted, and care was given by professionals in gowns, masks and visors. There is already research exploring the negative impact of these restrictions on aspects such as maternal mental health (Dib et al., 2020). A Europe-wide commentary by Lalor et al. (2021) argued that many of the measures brought in to keep women, babies and staff safe went against the need to preserve human rights in pregnancy and birth. In terms of communication, the challenge of supporting women while wearing a mask or visor is obvious—we rely on facial expressions as much as what we say, and the experience of being physically separate from those we are caring for affects us both. However, these short-term challenges might have longer-term effects—women's and families' experience of pregnancy and birth during COVID-19 may have long-term impacts on their mental health and wellbeing. Women may be more anxious in subsequent pregnancies, and potentially in need of a greater level of support than might otherwise be the case. We need to be aware of care and communication needs going forward.

A final point to consider in relation to communication is that birthing partners—who had gradually been welcomed into labour rooms from the late 1960s—suddenly found themselves shut out on the grounds of safety. As caregivers, we believe that we are offering 'family-centred care', but at the height of the pandemic we were doing anything but. In terms of communication, we need to make sure that partners are included in conversations and discussions and not left out because care takes place over the phone or via text message or because it feels safer to leave them in a corridor (see Vasilevskia et al., 2022, for a discussion about the experiences of partners and support persons during the pandemic in Australia).

## VIRTUAL COMMUNICATION

By reducing face-to-face contact and relying more heavily on phone or virtual communication, COVID-19 hastened changes already underway in terms of how we communicate with women and families. Some remote or rural areas of the world have always made use of telemedicine (telemedicine means using non-face-to-face means to give care), but the majority of people have only known in-person appointments with GPs, midwives or consultants.

For some people the move towards more virtual care might be positive. It can be more flexible and might allow for more open and relaxed communication than in a formal appointment situation. However, some people may struggle with the lack of personal contact—particularly groups who are already disadvantaged due to poverty, ethnicity, lack of access to telephone or Internet, or who do not easily communicate in English. The challenge will be to consider individual needs when planning and delivering communication in maternity, and to remember how multifaceted and complex good communication can be to provide.

An example of changing communication is the growing use of digital maternity notes. These systems have the advantage of documenting care across all health professionals in one place—they can include scan and other test results, notes by midwives, doctors and support workers to name a few. Antenatal, postnatal and labour notes are together and they cannot be lost or misinterpreted due to poor handwriting or the use of nonuniversal acronyms. Women can access their own notes, which should help to make care communication more responsive and open. The Ockenden Report calls for the continued development of digital notes as a key component of safer maternity care (Ockenden, 2022, p. 161). We need to be careful, however, to continue to prioritise confidentiality and to ensure that women as individuals do not get lost in a system of drop-down menus and space to record only certain information.

The Royal College of Midwives in the UK has published information about undertaking effective virtual consultations. They make some key points about ensuring good practice.

---

**PRACTICE POINTS**

Effective virtual consultations:
- Consider individual circumstances and the nature of the appointment. Is it appropriate to be virtual?
- Offer a choice of virtual or in-person where possible.
- Consider privacy—particularly when discussing sensitive topics.
- Be aware of the need for clear documentation, including whether the consultation was via telephone, video or face to face.

Adapted from RCM. (2021). *Giving virtual consultations in maternity*. https://www.rcm.org.uk/news-views/news/2020/giving-virtual-consultations-in-maternity/

Individual appointments are not the only way that midwives can connect with women and families during the childbearing year. In Chapter 14, we explored how midwives might use social media to develop professional connections and build knowledge. It can also be used to develop virtual communities of care—either alongside or in place of in-person encounters such as antenatal groups. There are positives to using this approach; people might be more open, it can give opportunities for peer support to develop and it can be effective in reaching a larger number of people effectively. However, some people may be unwilling or unable to use social media, and always, issues of confidentially and safeguarding need to be carefully considered in any online communication, even if the group is a closed, members-only one.

Finally, it is important that we pay attention to the impact that the move to virtual care has on us as health care professionals. Generally speaking, people join a profession such as midwifery because they enjoy working with people. Relationship building and communication are key facets of the role. We are used to giving personal care and support, whether to a person struggling with breast-feeding, someone anxious about test results or someone who wants to share the pride and joy of their birth experience. Having these conversations virtually is a new experience and given that this is likely to be the future of at least some aspects of care, we need to consider how to safeguard our own wellbeing and understanding of ourselves as professionals.

## THE FUTURE OF MIDWIFERY

This very short section cannot discuss exhaustively all the ways that the midwifery profession and midwifery care might evolve in the future. It simply aims to highlight a few issues where communication has a particular impact.

**COFFEE BREAK ACTIVITY**

Jot down a few bullet points outlining what you think midwifery practice will look like in 2030.
 Think about:
1. Midwifery education
2. Place of work
3. Organisation of care
4. Relationships to other professionals
5. Relationships with pregnant people and families
6. Effect of medical and technical advances
7. Social and political issues that might have an impact

- How will our skills, knowledge and practice around communication change to support these developments?
- What core skills in communication will remain important?

As this book was being written, the Ockenden Report was published. This report looked into poor care and outcomes at the Shrewsbury and Telford Hospitals between 2000 and 2020, although some cases went back as far as 1973. The Report has been referenced throughout this book. Its recommended actions include more time for training and updating, more robust and responsive investigation processes and a move away from the monitoring of Caesarean section rates (with the implication that lower was better), and these have been discussed at appropriate points in this book (Ockenden, 2022, see Chapter 15). Its specific recommendations will have a concrete impact on midwifery, but also a wider impact in relation to beliefs and attitudes. The Report follows the *Kirkup Report* (Kirkup, 2015) and *Better Births* (NHS England, 2017) in foregrounding safety and team working as essential elements of a modern service. Concepts such as 'normal birth' and being 'with woman' which were once cornerstones of midwifery philosophy and practice are now seen as complex and potentially problematic. Midwives need to understand contemporary discussions around the organisation of care and consider where they fit into practice. For most practitioners this is likely to revolve around enhanced team working. Looking forward, it is also vital that we remain open to debate and challenge, and humble in the face of what families tell us they want and need from maternity services and from midwives. Open, honest and respectful communication will continue to help us as we negotiate the challenges of 21st century midwifery practice.

## Conclusion

This chapter has considered the individual midwifery practitioner. It has explored how we communicate, and how reflection, support and goal setting can be used in building our personal practice toolkit. Finally, it has discussed briefly some of the challenges of contemporary practice, including COVID-19, virtual communication and the future of midwifery. These have been put into the context of how we continue to develop our communication, ensuring that it is dynamic, responsive and meaningful.

### References

Austin, D., Gilkison, A., & Clemons, J. (2020). Turning reflection into learning: A practice development tool for midwifery students. *Reflective Practice*, *21*(3), 301–315.

Bass, J., Fenwick, J., & Sidebotham, M. (2017). Development of a model of holistic reflection to facilitate transformative learning in student midwives. *Women and Birth*, *30*, 227–235.

Brown, T., Williams, B., Boyle, M., Molloy, M., McKenna, L., Palermo, C., Molloy, L., & Lewis, B. (2011). Communication styles of undergraduate health students. *Nurse Education Today*, *31*, 317–322.

Dib, S., Rougeaux, E., Vázquez-Vázquez, A., Wells, J., & Fewtrell, M. (2020). Maternal mental health and coping during the COVID-19 lockdown in the UK: Data from the COVID-19 New Mum Study. *International Journal of Gynaecology and Obstetrics*, *151*, 407–414. https://doi.org/10.1002/ijgo.13397.

Kirkham, M. (1997). Reflection in midwifery: Professional narcissism or seeing with women? *British Journal of Midwifery, 5*(5), 259–262.

Kirkup, B. *Morecombe Bay investigation: Report.* 2015. https://www.gov.uk/government/publications/morecambe-bay-investigation-report

Lalor, J., Ayers, S., Celleja Agius, J., Downe, S., Gouni, O., Hartmann, K., Nieuwenhuijze, M., Oosterman, M., Turner, J. D., Karlsdottir, S. I., & Horschk, A. (2021). Balancing restrictions and access to maternity care for women and birthing partners during the COVID-19 pandemic: The psychosocial impact of suboptimal care. *BJOG, 128,* 1720–1725.

McIntosh, T. (2012). *A social history of maternity care.* Routledge.

McKenzie, P. J. (2010). Informing relationships: Small talk, informing and relationship building in midwife-woman interaction. *Information Research, 15*(1), 423. http://InformationR.net/ir/15-1/paper423.html.

NHS England. *Better births: National maternity review.* 2017. national-maternity-review-report.pdf (https://england.nhs.uk)

NHS England. *A-EQUIP: A model of clinical midwifery supervision.* 2017. https://www.england.nhs.uk/publication/a-equip-a-model-of-clinical-midwifery-supervision/

NMC. *Standards of proficiency for midwives.* 2019. https://www.nmc.org.uk/standards/standards-for-midwives/standards-of-proficiency-for-midwives/

Norton, R. W. (1978). Foundation of a communicator style construct. *Human Communication Research, 4*(2), 99–112.

Ockenden, D. (2022). *Ockenden report – final: Findings, conclusions and essential actions from the Independent Review of Maternity Services at The Shrewsbury and Telford Hospital NHS Trust.* Her Majesty's Stationery Office (HMSO). https://assets.publishing.service.gov.uk/government/uploads/system/uploads/attachment_data/file/1064302/Final-Ockenden-Report-web-accessible.pdf.

Vasilevski, V., Sweet, L., Bradfield, Z., Wilson, A. N., Hauck, Y., Kuliukas, L., Homer, C., Szabo, R. A., & Wynter, K. (2022). Receiving maternity care during the COVID-19 pandemic: Experiences of women's partners and support persons. *Women and Birth, 35,* 298–306. http://doi.org/10.1016/j.wombi.2021.04.012.

Wain, A. (2017). Learning through reflection. *British Journal of Midwifery, 25*(10), 662–666.

## Resources

Godfrey-Issacs, L. (2020). *'Hello, can you hear me' – virtual midwifery in a pandemic.* https://www.all4maternity.com/hello-can-you-hear-me-virtual-midwifery-in-a-pandemic/?sfw=pass1649251067

*Godfrey-Issacs, a midwife and artist, has written a thoughtful and personal article about the experience of providing community midwifery care in the UK during the COVID-19 pandemic.*

RCM. (2021). *Giving virtual consultations in maternity.* https://www.rcm.org.uk/news-views/news/2020/giving-virtual-consultations-in-maternity

*The RCM has produced a document and poster giving midwives practical advice on planning and managing virtual consultations during the childbearing year.*

Wain, A. (2017). Learning through reflection. *British Journal of Midwifery, 25*(10), 662–666.

*This paper is a clear explanation of the main reflective models used in midwifery practice.*

# CHAPTER 16

# Conclusion

Tania Staras

The idea for this book came from my years of experience as a midwife and researcher and as a teacher of student midwives. There are so many wonderful resources available on midwifery practice: textbooks, research papers, internet blogs and videos. However, it felt to me that there was a gap when it came to specific information and ideas about communication in midwifery. Maybe that is because communication is so central to midwifery practice that we assume that we will know about it and understand it. This book has tried not to make that assumption—it explores the range of midwifery practice but puts communication at the heart of every discussion.

We all have knowledge and skills when it comes to communication—we use it every day in every situation and have done since the day we were born. For this reason, perhaps, we can feel that we can easily translate our day-to-day practice into our professional role. To a certain extent of course we can—our human empathy, kindness and care, our ability to listen, speak, read and write are all central to our practice as midwives. This book has taken our core understanding of communication and built on it. Different chapters have explored communication across the childbearing year, in challenging circumstances and with the multidisciplinary team. We have considered theories and histories of communication and the different ways we can use it—not just face to face or through writing, but also through developing forms such as social media and creativity.

Hopefully this book has introduced you to new ideas and given you evidence and information that build your theoretical understanding of communication in midwifery. As you will have seen, however, it is also a very practical book. Each chapter is full of short exercises, reflections, case studies and practice points. You can use the book to develop a portfolio of evidence and reflection around your communication practice. In this way, you can actively shape your own toolkit of skills and ideas which are applicable to you in your practice.

Inevitability in an edited collection such as this, there are some areas of repetition. This is partly because every element of the book is interlinked. If you have picked up this book to dip into one chapter, you may find that it leads you to explore others. Let's take the labour chapter as an example:

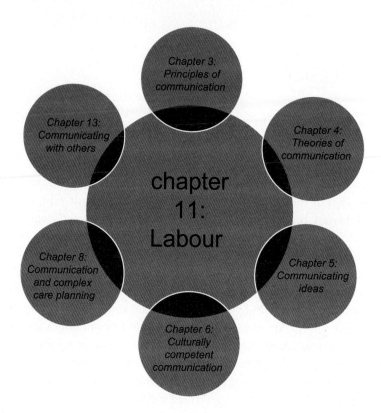

As you can see in the diagram, the chapter on communication during labour and birth can be read as complete in itself. However, the ideas and issues in the chapter are related to those found in other chapters which might be worth exploring to develop your ideas. Depending on your area of interest you might include other chapters in this diagram—perhaps the one on public health (Chapter 7) or on loss and trauma (Chapter 9). Each chapter takes a particular area of focus and guides you and challenges you as you work through it. You will have seen that there are key ideas and principles that are relevant throughout regardless of the specific issue or element of the childbearing journey.

**COFFEE BREAK ACTIVITY**

Make a quick bullet-point list of key things you have learned from this book.

# Key Ideas and Principles

The one key principle of this book was first mentioned in the Introduction (Chapter 1):

*And always remember that good communication is not an optional extra in midwifery—it is midwifery.*

As this book has tried to demonstrate, 'good communication' is not one simple skill that can be learned and used in all situations. It is individual and dynamic—depending on you, the person or people you are communicating with, the situation and the medium you are using to communicate. The practicalities of communicating with a newly pregnant adolescent who has English as a second language will be different to escalating your concerns about a pathological cardiotocograph (CTG) to an obstetric colleague. Nevertheless, there are key principles in each case:

- **Listen**. Pay attention to what the other person is communicating but also be aware of nonverbal cues such as tone of voice and body language.
- **Check**. Is your communication clear—does the other person genuinely understand what you are trying to get across?
- **Give space**. Communication works best when there is an exchange rather than when one person is transmitting, and the other person is receiving. When you are communicating, leave space in your communication for the other person to absorb and process information, and to add to it and ask questions.
- **Don't make assumptions**. It's easy to assume that others have heard and understood what you have said/written and the context of your communication. Be aware of the complexity of language but also of cultural assumptions. When listening to others, don't assume that you understand what they are trying to get across.
- **Be kind and respectful**. A lot of communication in midwifery can seem very routine. It might be routine for health professionals, but it isn't for women, birthing people and families. Think about what you say, how you say it, and how it comes across to people who might be confused, excited, anxious, scared or sad.
- **See everyone as an individual**. Treat everyone and every encounter as an individual experience.
- **Be flexible**. People change their minds and their opinions and that's ok. We change and develop and so do practice situations. Use flexibility in your communication and remember that no idea or plan is set in stone.
- **Be honest**. If things aren't going to plan or outcomes are complex or uncertain, then communicate this sensitively and honestly. Don't be afraid to admit to mistakes and to apologise. People can cope better with difficult and challenging experiences if the communication is clear, unambiguous and open.

There may be others that you would add because of your experience and your reading of this book.

# A Final Thought

As we have said throughout this book, communication is at the heart of midwifery practice. It matters to the people in our care, and it matters to our colleagues and to the service and to society generally. Families remember less about the clinical details of care and more about how they were spoken to, how things were explained to them and ultimately whether they were genuinely listened to.

Hopefully you have been able to use this book to explore communication in midwifery and as a springboard to developing and deepening your knowledge and skills in this vital area.

Note: Page numbers followed by *f* indicate figures, *t* indicate tables, and *b* indicate boxes.